Getting Started as a

Pharmacy Faculty
Member

Notice

The author, editor, and publisher have made every effort to ensure the accuracy and completeness of the information presented in this book. However, the author, editor, and publisher cannot be held responsible for the continued currency of the information, any inadvertent errors or omissions, or the application of this information. Therefore, the author, editor, and publisher shall have no liability to any person or entity with regard to claims, loss, or damage caused or alleged to be caused, directly or indirectly, by the use of information contained herein.

Getting Started as a
Pharmacy Faculty Member

David P. Zgarrick, BPharm, PhD

Professor and Chair
Department of Pharmacy Practice
School of Pharmacy
Bouvé College of Health Sciences
Northeastern University
Boston, Massachusetts

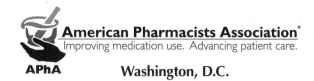

American Pharmacists Association®
Improving medication use. Advancing patient care.

APhA   Washington, D.C.

Managing and Content Editor: Vicki Meade, Meade Communications
Acquiring Editor: Julian Graubart
Proofreader: Amy Morgante
Indexer: Lisa McInnis, Columbia Indexing Group
Cover Designer: Scott Neitzke, APhA Creative Services
Layout and Graphics: Michele A. Danoff, Graphics by Design

© 2010 by the American Pharmacists Association
APhA was founded in 1852 as the American Pharmaceutical Association.

Published by the American Pharmacists Association
2215 Constitution Avenue, N.W.
Washington, DC 20037-2985
www.pharmacylibrary.com   www.pharmacist.com

To comment on this book via email, send your message to the publisher at
aphabooks@aphanet.org.

Library of Congress Cataloging-in-Publication Data

Zgarrick, David P.
  Getting started as a pharmacy faculty member / by David P. Zgarrick.
     p. ; cm.
  Includes bibliographical references and index.
  ISBN 978-1-58212-149-9
  1. Pharmacy colleges—Faculty—Vocational guidance. 2.
Pharmacy—Study and teaching. I. American Pharmacists Association. II.
Title.
  [DNLM: 1. Education, Pharmacy—United States. 2. Faculty—United States.
3. Vocational Guidance—United States. QV 19]
  RS101.Z53 2010
  615'.1023—dc22
                         2010027168

How to Order This Book

Online: www.pharmacist.com/shop_apha
By phone: 800-878-0729 (from the United States and Canada)
VISA®, MasterCard®, and American Express® cards accepted

Contents

Preface

Welcome to *Getting Started as a Pharmacy Faculty Member*. Anyone reading this book is likely to be considering a career in academia. Many student pharmacists, residents, research fellows, and graduate students think about career paths in academia, as do experienced pharmacists and other professionals. If you fall into any of these groups, you probably have a lot of questions about just what this career entails and what it takes to be successful.

Or maybe you've already embarked on a career in academic pharmacy and are wondering, like many of us have at some point, "Just what have I gotten myself into?" This book should help clarify what lies ahead.

The purpose of this book is to help you learn more about careers in academic pharmacy and set a course for a successful career. Many people in academic pharmacy, including me, did not know much of what this book reveals before we started our careers. We knew how to be a student, resident, fellow, or graduate student, but the experience of a faculty member is much different.

We developed successful careers anyway, to some extent through trial and error, but any seasoned faculty member will tell you that the more you know before starting your career, the better choices you are likely to make as your career progresses. And the first of all those choices is deciding whether a career in academic pharmacy is right for you.

This book is structured chronologically as much as possible, starting with a chapter about why you should consider a career in academic pharmacy. The second chapter delves into the nature of the work of a professor at a college of pharmacy, which varies depending on the position and the college's expectations—but almost all of the work can be categorized as teaching, scholarship, or service.

The third chapter explores the way colleges and universities function. You'll learn about the different types of academic institutions and appointments, how universities and colleges of pharmacy are structured, and where you fit in as a new faculty member. You'll also get insights into how colleges and universities operate, how decisions are made at a variety of levels, and the role of faculty members in governing an institution and making decisions.

Once you've decided to pursue an academic career, you'll want to boost the chances that you'll obtain a position aligned with your interests and goals. The fourth and fifth chapters cover what it takes to navigate through the academic employment process. As with any professional position, the process of seeking a faculty appointment is quite competitive. The more you know about searching, applying, and interviewing, the more likely you will be to get the position you want and to start your academic career on the right path.

A key message I want to convey is that there is no single correct way to achieve success in academic pharmacy. For this reason, Chapter 6 includes interviews with five pharmacists who've navigated their way to rewarding careers as faculty members. These pharmacists came to academia from a variety of backgrounds and each holds different types of positions, ranging from laboratory research scientist to ambulatory care clinical practitioner. They all work for universities with distinctly diverse missions. Despite these differences, you'll see that these five professors have a great deal in common. Much can be learned from their experiences to help you move in the right direction for a bright future in academic pharmacy.

The last two chapters provide practical advice for starting your career and resources that offer guidance and answer questions. As a faculty member and administrator at the midpoint of my career, I've included in Chapter 7 my own insights about achieving success in academic pharmacy.

Although launching your career is challenging, most pharmacists and professionals who have pursued careers as faculty at colleges of pharmacy will tell you that the rewards outweigh the challenges. Every time I meet a student pharmacist, resident, research fellow, or graduate student who is interested in academia, I'm reminded of my own feelings as I started planning my future. I felt a little hesitant, based on things I'd heard about academia, but I discovered that most of it was misinformation. Ultimately, I was drawn to an academic career by my passion for teaching, research, and serving my colleagues, profession, and the public.

Many pharmacy careers have the potential to be professionally satisfying. But I know of no other that gives you as much control over how you define yourself as being a faculty member at a college of pharmacy.

David P. Zgarrick
June 2010

Acknowledgments

This project would have been impossible without the support of many people who played a role in my development as a faculty member. The list is so long, I hesitate to mention people by name because I'm afraid I'll leave someone out, but I'm thankful to everyone who played a role in my development or helped make this book possible.

Like many others in academic pharmacy, I didn't start my career thinking I'd be a faculty member and administrator. While I was getting my BS in pharmacy at the University of Wisconsin – Madison, I had the good fortune to interact with faculty members in the classroom, performing research, on committees, and in a variety of professional organizations, giving me a well-rounded sense of what they do. They taught me that their work was not only interesting and challenging, but also a lot of fun. I'll always be grateful for their influence and encouragement as I started down my career path.

My development continued as a graduate student at The Ohio State University College of Pharmacy, where I gained experience as a teacher—which was exciting as well as humbling—and as a researcher. The faculty at Ohio State continued to nurture me as I progressed toward the beginning of my academic career.

My first academic appointment was at Midwestern University Chicago College of Pharmacy (MWU). MWU had just started a pharmacy school when I joined their faculty, which in and of itself gave me unique opportunities to develop as a new faculty member. But I never would have been able to take advantage of those opportunities if it weren't for the students, staff, faculty colleagues, and especially my first department chair. Their willingness to share their knowledge and experience played an invaluable role in my development.

I'd also like to thank my colleagues at Drake University, who helped me grow as an administrator. Finally, thank you to my current colleagues at Northeastern University, who have been patient with me as I adapt to yet another new university and administrative position while writing this book.

The American Pharmacists Association (APhA) is providing a great service to pharmacists by developing this series of "Getting Started" guides. I'd like to thank the APhA leaders who had the foresight to include *Getting Started as a Pharmacy Faculty Member* in the series and recommend me as an author. In particular, I'd like to thank Julian Graubart and Vicki Meade for their advice and encouragement as I developed this book. Thanks also to the five faculty members who generously volunteered time to share their experiences in Chapter 6. For reviewing a draft of this book, my thanks to Andrea Kjos, PharmD, PhD, assistant professor of pharmacy administration at Drake University, and Janis MacKichan, PharmD, vice chair and professor of pharmacy practice at Northeast Ohio Universities College of Pharmacy.

Most important, thanks go to my family, and especially my wife, Michelle Zgarrick, PharmD, who has been my friend and confidante throughout my career. She lived through everything I experienced as a faculty member and was a sounding board for practically every idea you're reading about in this book. As a pharmacist, Michelle helps me stay grounded in the profession and reminds me just how important the work of pharmacy faculty is to all the groups we serve: students, pharmacists, other health professionals, patients, and society at large. I can't imagine this book, or my career, being possible without her support.

Dedication

To my teachers, mentors, colleagues, and students.

Chapter 1

Is an Academic Career a Good Fit for You?

Of all of the career paths you can follow in pharmacy, why would you want to be a faculty member at a college of pharmacy? It's a fair question, with many good answers.

According to the American Pharmacists Association's Career Pathway Evaluation Program for Pharmacy Professionals, several themes recur among the clinical practitioners, pharmaceutical scientists, and economic, social, and administrative scientists who pursue careers in academic pharmacy. These professionals enjoy:

- **Teaching and working with student pharmacists.** Nothing keeps you "young at heart" more than interacting with a group of students.

- **Learning.** They have an inquisitive nature. Academia appeals to the type of pharmacist who, when presented with a new issue or problem, immediately wonders, "Why or how did this issue come to be?" or "What can we do now that would be better than what was done in the past?" Academic pharmacists enjoy the challenge of staying on top of new knowledge in their fields, especially when it comes to working with students.

- **Solving problems through innovative thinking.** They often design experiments and collect data to evaluate the value of each new approach, whether they are in the laboratory, clinic, hospital, pharmacy, or classroom.

- **Variety.** They seek positions that require them to perform a diverse range of activities, from giving lectures and precepting students to carrying out research and serving on committees. They are comfortable handling multiple tasks, often at the same time.

- **Autonomy and flexibility**. Academic pharmacists are self-directed and like to set their own schedules regarding where and when they perform their work.

- **Working in teams.** Pharmacists in academia work with others in a variety of ways, such as teaching in teams in the classroom, serving on committees that provide direction to their organizations, and performing research and other scholarly projects that discover, integrate, and apply knowledge.

- **Prestige.** Professionals in academia are held in high esteem by pharmacists, other health care professionals, and the community in general.

Academicians recognize that their careers may not offer the highest salaries in the profession, especially at the entry level, but they realize that their careers come with many tangible and intangible benefits, such as those cited above. Most faculty members feel that the value of these benefits more than makes up for the difference in salary they could earn in other settings.

Many Roles Outside the Classroom

A professor lecturing to students from the front of the classroom is usually the first, and often the only, image that comes to mind when we think about a faculty member. Although teaching is an essential function for most college of pharmacy faculty, you can hold many other positions that may or may not put you at the head of a classroom full of students. These include:

> Nothing keeps you "young at heart" more than interacting with a group of students.

- **Administrators** such as deans, assistant and associate deans, department chairs, and program directors.

- **Research scientists** who work in laboratories, clinics, and offices.

- **Experiential education specialists** who identify, develop, and evaluate practice sites and preceptors suitable for introductory pharmacy practice experiences (IPPEs) and advanced pharmacy practice experiences (APPEs).

- **Laboratory instructors** who assist students as they acquire the knowledge and skills necessary to practice.

- **Pharmacy practitioners** who serve as preceptors for students undergoing IPPEs and APPEs.

In later chapters, this book will provide more information on the background and qualifications necessary to pursue a position at a college of pharmacy. Most of these positions require additional education and training beyond the doctor of pharmacy (PharmD) degree, but some do not.

The Demand Continues

Pharmacy faculty will continue to be in demand. Society needs pharmacists with an ever-broadening scope of practice, especially in the area of patient care. Yet society can't begin to meet the demand for pharmacists without a sufficient number of colleges of pharmacy and, most important, without the faculty members to teach pharmacy students. Drug therapy is an ever-increasing aspect of health care, with the number of prescriptions filled in the United States more than doubling between 1995 and 2010. And legislation such as the Medicare Prescription Drug, Improvement, and Modernization Act of 2003 (Medicare Part D) and the Patient Protection and Affordable Care Act of 2010 (Health Care Reform) expands the pool of people with access to prescription medications, medication therapy management, and other clinical services that pharmacists provide.

As the "Baby Boom" generation born between the mid-1940s and mid-1960s reaches retirement, the demand for pharmaceuticals, pharmacists' clinical services, and pharmacy education is certain to grow.

According to the American Association of Colleges of Pharmacy (AACP), the number of colleges of pharmacy, first professional degree students, and faculty members have all increased substantially since 1990 (see Figure 1-1). Projections by the U.S. Health Resources and Services Administration (HRSA) Adequacy of Pharmacist Supply Report show that the demand for pharmacists and pharmacy services will continue to increase as the population grows, ages, and increasingly relies on medications to manage both acute and chronic health conditions.

While the increased number of pharmacy schools, faculty, and graduates has helped to address shortages that existed earlier in the decade, projections indicate that the demand for pharmacists, as well as for colleges of pharmacy and faculty members, will remain high. Figures 1-2 and 1-3 show how the numbers of pharmacy faculty and students increased over the two decades surrounding the turn of the 21st century.

Figure 1-1 | **Number of Schools of Pharmacy - 1990–2009**

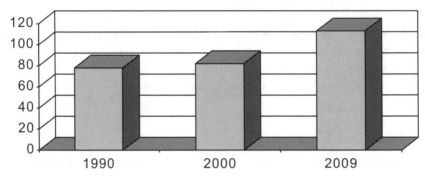

Source: American Association of Colleges of Pharmacy

Figure 1-2 | **First Professional Degree Students - 1990–2009**

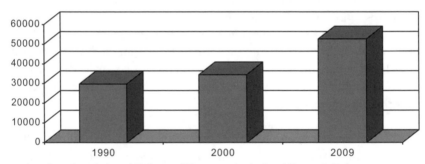

Source: American Association of Colleges of Pharmacy, Institutional Research Data
(www.aacp.org/resources/research/institutionalresearch)

Figure 1-3 | **Number of Full-Time Pharmacy Faculty - 1990–2009**

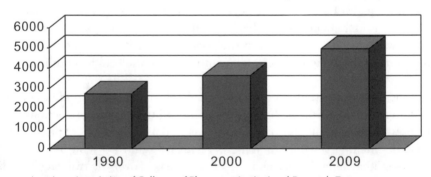

Source: American Association of Colleges of Pharmacy, Institutional Research Data
(www.aacp.org/resources/research/institutionalresearch)

Implications for You

What does this ongoing need for pharmacists mean for you? The keys to a long and enjoyable career in any field involve not only continued demand for particular services, but also for a set of knowledge and skills necessary to achieve success. If you are interested in academia, you should have many opportunities, because new pharmacists need to be recruited and trained on an ongoing basis. And as medical knowledge and pharmacy practice evolve, pharmacy educators will be on the forefront of discovering new knowledge and educating both patients and students. This requires pharmacy educators to continue learning themselves.

> Professionals in academia are held in high esteem by pharmacists, other health care professionals, and the community in general.

The remainder of this guide will provide information about what college professors are expected to do, how universities and colleges are structured and operate, and steps you'll need to take to start down the path toward a career in academic pharmacy. You'll get advice from successful faculty members from a variety of backgrounds.

Finally, you will learn what you can do to ease your transition into the role of a pharmacy faculty member and discover resources available to help you achieve success. Pharmacy faculty members who reviewed this book before publication said it contains details they wish they'd known before starting their careers. I hope it gives you knowledge at the start of your career that others had to gain by trial and error later on.

Where to Find More Information on Attributes of and Demand for Pharmacy Educators

American Pharmacists Association (APhA) Career Pathway Evaluation Program for Pharmacy Professionals
www.pharmacist.com
This program provides resources that allow pharmacists to assess their own interests and then learn about careers in pharmacy matching those interests. Many colleges of pharmacy offer the program as a live workshop

continued on page 6

continued from page 5

for their students. Interested students and pharmacists can also access the materials online at the URL above and search the Career Pathway Evaluation Program section.

American Association of Colleges of Pharmacy (AACP) – Academic Pharmacy's Vital Statistics

www.aacp.org/about/Pages/Vitalstats.aspx
AACP regularly gathers data from U.S. colleges of pharmacy, including the numbers of students enrolled in their programs, the types of programs they offer, the number and type of faculty members employed, and annual salary and benefit trends.

Health Resources and Services Administration (HRSA) Adequacy of Pharmacist Supply Report

http://bhpr.hrsa.gov/healthworkforce/pharmacy/supplyadequacy.htm
This report presents the results of a study performed by the U.S. Department of Health and Human Services in 2004 assessing the adequacy of pharmacist services and identifying trends likely to impact demand for these services up to 2030.

Pharmacy Manpower Project

www.pharmacymanpower.com
The Pharmacy Manpower Project (PMP) collects, analyzes, and disseminates information on the supply and demand for licensed pharmacists in the U.S. A key component of the PMP website is the Aggregate Demand Index (ADI), which collects data from a panel of pharmacy employers to track changes in pharmacist supply and demand across practice settings and regions on a monthly basis.

Chapter 2

Academic Pharmacy's "Big Three"

Now that you're thinking about getting started as a pharmacy faculty member, it's likely you've tried to answer the question, "What exactly does a faculty member at a college of pharmacy do?"

Based on your experience as a student, you already know that faculty teach in various venues, including classrooms, laboratories, and clinical practice sites. But is teaching as simple as lecturing to students about what the faculty member knows or telling students in a lab or practice site what they should or shouldn't do? And what activities do pharmacy faculty members engage in when they're not teaching? A popular misconception is that when faculty members are not in the classroom or at their practice site they are on vacation or taking a break. But if you ask them, you'll learn that's definitely *not* the case.

The Academic Triad

Virtually everything that a faculty member does at any college or university is captured by three categories within what is known as the "academic triad":

- Teaching
- Scholarship
- Service

Every academic institution sets different expectations, and faculty members at some colleges may concentrate most on one or two of the activities. For example, some colleges expect their faculty to spend more time teaching, while some place more emphasis on research and other forms of scholarship.

If you're a clinical preceptor or laboratory instructor, it's likely that you are only involved in teaching. Most pharmacy faculty members, however, must take part in the entire triad to be successful. It can be challenging to spread yourself out over three different types of activities, but it's a challenge that attracts many people to careers in academia instead of other areas of pharmacy.

This chapter provides details on the triad of activities in which pharmacy faculty are involved. My purpose in this chapter is not to tell you how to be a good teacher, scholar, or service provider, but rather to give you a better appreciation for everything a pharmacy faculty member does, both "on stage" and "behind the scenes."

> Most pharmacy faculty have an ardent love for learning, and learning is inherent in all good teaching.

Teaching

On the surface, teaching appears to be a relatively simple, straightforward activity, especially for trained professionals who have a wealth of useful knowledge, such as pharmacists. After all, at its most basic level, teaching involves transferring knowledge from an expert, such as a college professor or a pharmacist, to a learner, such as a student pharmacist or patient. The key, however, is knowing how to *effectively* transfer knowledge so learners can understand and apply it. Teaching is a skill that is harder than it looks.

Most pharmacy faculty have an ardent love for learning, and learning is inherent in all good teaching. Teachers can't teach concepts that they haven't first learned themselves. And because pharmacy, the biomedical sciences, and the health care environment are constantly changing, the best teachers are constantly learning.

Teaching Methods

One of the first challenges teachers face is determining the most appropriate ways to transfer knowledge to their students. During the many years you have spent as a learner, you've gained knowledge in several different ways and you know that some methods of teaching are more effective for you than others. And you recognize that what works best depends on the nature of the material you are learning.

You probably find that reading a book or listening to a lecture works well for learning some material, but sometimes hands-on application is more useful. Certainly you've noticed that peers and classmates differ in their learning preferences. For example, you might read a book chapter and find the concepts crystal clear, while some classmates who read the same chapter feel confused by the material.

Because students have different learning styles and because pharmacy involves such diverse skills and concepts, pharmacy faculty must use a variety of teaching methods, including:

- **Lecturing.** Most people associate teaching with the traditional "on stage" lecture in which faculty transmit information to students using primarily one-way communication. Pharmacy faculty provide lectures in settings ranging from large auditorium-style classrooms with an audience of hundreds to small classes with a handful of students.

- **Facilitating seminars.** Many pharmacy faculty facilitate sessions in which a small group of students explore a specific topic. These sessions rely heavily on a two-way exchange of ideas between the faculty member and students.

- **Facilitating laboratory sessions.** Some pharmacy faculty teach by creating and facilitating activities that students perform in a laboratory, which allows students to apply what they have learned and practice skills that they will later use in real-life practice. Areas that lend themselves to laboratory facilitation include applied sciences (e.g., chemistry, biology), pharmaceutical sciences (e.g., pharmaceutics, pharmacokinetics), pharmacy practice (e.g., compounding, medication preparation, order processing, and dispensing), patient communications, physical assessment, medication therapy management, drug information, and pharmacy practice management.

- **Meeting with students.** A great deal of teaching occurs outside the classroom or laboratory. Students commonly make appointments to see faculty members during office hours to discuss topics that they either didn't understand or would like to learn about in greater depth. Pharmacy faculty also meet with students to advise them on a number of matters, including helping them learn more about career options and professional development opportunities.

- **Precepting.** Almost a third of the doctor of pharmacy curriculum consists of experiences in which faculty supervise students as they learn how pharmacists practice. While most introductory pharmacy practice experiences (IPPEs) and advanced pharmacy practice experiences (APPEs) occur in patient care settings, they can take place anywhere that pharmacists work, such as pharmacy professional organizations, hospital or chain pharmacy administrative offices, and government agencies. Some pharmacy faculty offer rotations in their laboratories and research settings; others offer teaching rotations in their classrooms to introduce students to the principles and practice of teaching and learning.

Pedagogical Skills

Being an effective teacher and facilitator of student learning takes special knowledge and skills, which are just as important as the knowledge and skills necessary to become an effective pharmacy practitioner. The knowledge, skills, and methods used to impart learning are commonly referred to as *pedagogy*.

Although many educators formally learned about pedagogy while they were in college, particularly those teaching at the K–12 level, most college professors—including pharmacy faculty members—are hired based on their clinical and research abilities, not their teaching skills. Pedagogy is something most pharmacy faculty members learn once they are on the job.

Fortunately, a number of resources are available to teach pharmacy faculty the pedagogical skills they need to be effective teachers. Many universities provide faculty development programs that review pedagogical techniques, often as part of their new faculty orientation programs. University-based programs typically give access to books, articles, and other learning resources, presentations on pedagogical technologies and techniques, and opportunities to learn from experienced teachers.

> The knowledge, skills, and methods used to impart learning are commonly referred to as pedagogy.

Colleges of pharmacy often have their own professional development programming to help faculty learn the specific types of teaching that best prepare students to become pharmacists. Several professional pharmacy associations have programs to help pharmacy faculty members develop and improve their teaching skills, including the Education Scholar Program offered by the American Association of Colleges of Pharmacy (AACP) and the American College of Clinical Pharmacy (ACCP) Academy Teaching and Learning Certificate Program.

Applying pedagogical skills and knowledge to teach effectively can be challenging and takes a great deal of time. Among the specific challenges are:

- **Preparation.** It's not unusual for a pharmacy faculty member to put many hours into preparing a single learning resource or presentation. Among specific tasks involved in preparing for effective teaching:
  o Reviewing existing knowledge and literature in the topic to be taught.
  o Determining important points that students should learn.
  o Preparing resources to be used in teaching, such as PowerPoint slides.
  o Developing materials students will use to learn, such as handouts and exercises.

- **Expectations.** Most pharmacy faculty are hired, at least in part, because of the expertise they have in their given fields. When it comes to teaching, faculty members must ask themselves, "What do these students need to know given where they are in their development?" and "How will they use this knowledge in the future?" Challenging students to learn and preparing them to apply knowledge later on are critical. Faculty should not, however, expect students to be at their own level of expertise, which is the result of many years of training and experience.

- **Pedagogical method.** Lectures are an efficient way to present or review large amounts of information in a short period of time, but they do not always promote effective student learning. Pharmacy faculty need to consider the nature of their material, the educational backgrounds of their students, and the way they expect students to learn and use the information. Our field involves such a vast amount of information that faculty need to tailor the methods they use to engage students, depending on the material, rather than lecturing to them all the time. Approaches may range from requiring students to read about a topic before class to employing discussions, group activities, and other active learning strategies.

- **Technology.** Technology has had a huge impact on how we teach and learn. Traditional lectures can become more interactive by using audience response technology or "clickers" to get immediate feedback. Entire courses can be recorded and put online for students to access from anywhere, anytime. Key challenges brought about by educational technology include deciding how and when to use it and understanding how to use it properly. Educational technology can be applied to any type of teaching, but pharmacy faculty must be judicious in its use. In many cases, the best opportunity for learning still involves direct interaction between learners and educators.

- **Assessment.** Pharmacy faculty must not only master teaching methods but also learn how to evaluate and give feedback to student pharmacists to promote their professional development. Most pharmacy faculty will tell you that student assessment is the most challenging aspect of teaching. On one hand, assessment is essential to learning. Students must be given constructive feedback to help them understand what they don't know as well as what they know. But assessment methods can be difficult to develop and evaluate. Despite the availability of professional development programs and other tools, learning how to develop valid assessments that correspond with specific objectives takes time, often as a result of much trial and error. Common assessment methods include:
  - Examinations (multiple choice items, calculations, essays)
  - Term papers
  - Projects
  - Objective structured clinical examinations (OSCEs)
  - Observations of performance on IPPEs and APPEs

Other Challenges

Many pharmacy faculty members are asked to coordinate entire courses or course sequences, which requires, at a minimum, a general understanding of the field being taught. The coordinator usually must decide:

- Which topics to cover?
- What level of detail will be involved?
- How will the topics be taught?
- How will student learning be assessed?

Course coordination also requires administrative skills related to scheduling, acquiring resources, understanding university and college policies, and providing feedback to other faculty and students.

Team-taught courses often present a unique challenge to new faculty members. Assigning multiple instructors to teach a particular course collaboratively is common today, given the breadth of topics covered in many pharmacy courses. The coordinator of team-taught courses must not only identify instructors with the necessary knowledge and background but also set and reinforce policies and standards, such as requiring all faculty to use a particular lecture format.

Instructors in team teaching situations must work closely with the coordinator to learn the course's overall objectives and needs. They often must adjust their individual styles and teaching methods for the sake of internal consistency across the course.

Scholarship

The words "research" and "scholarship" typically bring to mind images of people in white coats working in laboratories. Such work is critical to help us better understand diseases and develop therapies, but other, less apparent kinds of research that pharmacy faculty take part in are also important.

Evolution of Scholarship

The meaning of the word "scholarship" has evolved significantly over time. When universities were first developed in Europe during the Middle Ages, "scholarship" was used to broadly define the work of college professors. As recently as the 19th century, faculty scholarship consisted primarily of thinking, communicating (e.g., teaching), and learning. As universities entered the 20th century, they began to place more emphasis on creative efforts, particularly those related to creating new knowledge. In other words, "research" became a priority.

Because college professors are in the business of sharing their knowledge with students, a natural expectation at many universities was for professors to perform research to discover knowledge and then share that knowledge through publications, presentations, and teaching.

As universities evolved over the 20th century, they increasingly evaluated faculty members based on their research. At the same time, members of the public and some university administrators and faculty grew concerned about the impact this growing research emphasis was having on the value that universities placed on teaching.

Colleges of pharmacy also experienced changes during this time. In the early and middle 20th century, pharmacy education was primarily concerned with understanding the scientific underpinnings of how medications worked. Most pharmacy faculty had some role in researching and discovering knowledge about drugs while at the same time teaching student pharmacists how to prepare and dispense drugs to patients.

By the latter part of the 20th century, pharmacy education began to place more emphasis on understanding and teaching the clinical aspects of drug therapy. Student pharmacists were taught not only about the physical properties of medications they dispensed, but also how the actions of drugs impact patients and society. The role of the pharmacist ultimately began to change from a manufacturer and dispenser of a physical product to an information manager who works with other health professionals and patients to help them obtain the greatest benefit from drug therapy.

In addition to hiring faculty to research and teach about the physical aspects of drugs, colleges of pharmacy increasingly began to hire clinical faculty members who could research and teach about medications' effects on patients and society—working not just in laboratories on campus, but also in pharmacies, hospitals, and clinics where patients obtain or use medications.

Some pharmacy faculty, like faculty in other disciplines, struggled with the weight that universities placed on performing research. They perceived conflicts between their roles of discovering knowledge, teaching the next generation of professionals, and providing service to other health care providers and patients. Clinical practitioners in particular grew concerned about how their scholarly efforts would be evaluated, given the expectations placed on them to also care for patients and interact with other health professionals.

Types of Scholarship

Fortunately, through the work of Ernest Boyer and his colleagues with the Carnegie Foundation for the Advancement of Teaching, university administrators and faculty members were surveyed in the late 1980s to better understand how the emphasis on research was affecting the quality of undergraduate teaching. Recognizing that all college professors should be scholars, and that scholarship can take many forms, Boyer developed a paradigm in his classic book *Scholarship Reconsidered: Priorities of the Professoriate* that many universities adopted to redefine and broaden the scholarly expectations of their faculty. Boyer describes four different types of scholarly activity:

- **Scholarship of discovery.** This has to do with the search for knowledge for its own sake—commonly referred to as research. Although the modern world possesses a great body of knowledge, so much more is still unknown. Researchers apply the methods of scientific inquiry to continually seek out new knowledge. Pharmacy research can take many forms, including discovering new drugs, learning their mechanisms of action, developing new drug delivery methods, conducting clinical trials to understand a drug's safety and efficacy, and studying the social and economic implications of medication use.

- **Scholarship of integration.** Scholarship of discovery helps us gain new facts, but that does us little good unless we can place the facts in a broader perspective. Scholarship of integration takes facts discovered by researchers, both from within and across disciplines, and attempts to find relationships and connections to provide a better understanding of what these facts mean, how they can be applied to other contexts, and how they can refine the direction of future research.

A classic example of this type of scholarship is a project that evaluates the results of a number of studies and strives to interpret the combined findings. Clinical researchers have formalized such a process through a technique known as meta-analysis, in which the results of multiple studies are combined in a way that considers each study's methods, sample size, and results to reach a quantitative overall outcome.

- **Scholarship of application.** For outcomes of the previous two forms of scholarship to be useful in the real world, they must be able to be applied to problems we face. Those who engage in the scholarship of application—which is common for pharmacy faculty—seek to apply their knowledge and understanding of a field to solve problems at a variety of different levels.

Examples of the scholarship of application in pharmacy include chemists and pharmaceutics specialists who use their knowledge of nanotechnology to help a biotech company develop a new drug delivery system. A social scientist may use his knowledge of survey research to help a pharmacy association better understand an issue impacting its members. A pharmacist may apply her knowledge of drug therapy to solve problems for her patients and for other health professionals. An important aspect of the scholarship of application is using feedback and lessons learned to solve a particular problem. Scholars must recognize what works, as well as what doesn't, to better learn to solve problems in the future.

- **Scholarship of teaching.** By putting the previous three forms of scholarship together, Boyer recognized that the act of teaching, if done well, is inherently a scholarly activity. Teachers must be well informed in their fields, which commonly involves gaining significant amounts of knowledge (facts) and understanding the connections and relationships between them. Teachers must also understand and be able to describe how knowledge is used to solve problems. But above all, Boyer states, the act of teaching itself can be a focus of scholarship, particularly if teachers experiment with different forms of pedagogy and, using methods of scientific inquiry, investigate the impact of their teaching on outcomes important to their students—that is, learning.

Pharmacy faculty recognize that teaching is an important form of scholarship and they commonly experiment by using new forms of pedagogy in their teaching. They evaluate the outcomes of their teaching and share results in journals such as the *American Journal of Pharmaceutical Education* and *Currents in Pharmacy Teaching and Learning*.

Evaluating Scholarly Work

Scholarship is part of the academic triad described earlier and must be evaluated in terms of both quality and quantity, especially with respect to gaining promotion and tenure (see Chapter 3). Boyer spells out six standards by which all scholarly work should be evaluated:

- **Clear goals.** Each time you start a scholarly endeavor you should understand why you are performing the activity and what you hope to achieve.

- **Adequate preparation.** You should have an appropriate understanding of the issues you are investigating, problems you are solving, or disciplines in which you are teaching.

- **Appropriate methods.** You must understand and use methods appropriate to the task at hand.

- **Significant results.** The results of scholarly endeavors should create new knowledge, bring about a better understanding of existing knowledge, help solve a consequential problem, or help others better understand an issue.

- **Effective presentation.** For scholarship to be meaningful, it must be shared with others. This commonly begins with preparing an abstract or written report that is submitted to a panel of peers for critique and review. Once scholarship passes this level of review it can be presented as a written manuscript in a journal or as an oral presentation or poster at a conference. In this way, scholars create a forum to share what they have learned or done and to allow others the opportunity to further critique their findings, learn from their results, and apply what they've learned to their own scholarly efforts.

- **Reflective critique.** Scholars should look back at each endeavor to learn from their outcomes and from the methods and processes they used to achieve them. Most scholars will tell you that every scholarly project they embark upon commonly leads to asking more questions, which leads to additional scholarly projects. Scholars also use what they learn in their research to further inform and develop their teaching. This is commonly referred to as the teaching–research nexus.

> Scholars commonly use what they learn in their research to further inform and develop their teaching, which is called the "teaching–research nexus."

Service

You already knew that pharmacy faculty members were teachers, and you likely knew that most also perform some forms of scholarship. But are those activities enough to support the day-to-day operations of a university or a college of pharmacy? Don't college professors also have an obligation to make contributions and improvements to our profession, patients, and communities? Of course they do, which is why the third leg of the academic triad is service. Those outside of academia often don't think about service as part of the job of a pharmacy faculty member, but it is an essential component of the academic enterprise.

Although colleges and universities have administrative hierarchies similar to those in many workplaces, faculty members have a number of roles and responsibilities not commonly held by other employees. Most universities give the faculty members of each academic unit, such as the college of pharmacy, a wide range of powers to determine how their unit will operate.

Committees

Faculty and staff serve together on committees to shape operational and administrative functions. Most colleges of pharmacy have committees dealing with admissions, assessment, curriculum, student progression, promotion and tenure, scholarships, and awards, among many others. Through the committee structure, faculty members at most colleges of pharmacy take part in:

- Determining the curricula for their programs.
- Setting standards for the admission and progression of students through their programs.
- Deciding who will be hired as fellow faculty members.

- Developing criteria for evaluating whether a colleague should be promoted or receive tenure.

Committees are utilized at every level of the university, including the college and department levels. Most universities also have a faculty senate consisting of faculty members elected by their peers to develop university-wide policies and make recommendations to university administrators.

As a new pharmacy faculty member, it is likely that you will be assigned to a college of pharmacy committee soon after you start your position. The amount of time and effort you put into committee service depends on many factors. Administrators at some universities prefer that new faculty initially spend most of their time developing their teaching and scholarship, leaving committee service to more senior faculty. Other universities encourage new faculty to become active in committees as a way of socializing them into the operations of their academic units.

New faculty often have fewer responsibilities on committees than seasoned members do, which allows them to learn more about how the committee works and its role in the college's operations. Positions of leadership on college or university committees typically are filled by more experienced faculty, who set the agenda for what the committee will accomplish and interact with the constituencies it serves, such as other faculty, students, administrators, and alumni. If you are just getting started as a pharmacy faculty member, you will likely work with your department chair, dean, and other administrators to determine which committees you should serve on and what your level of involvement should be.

Patient Care

If you are a faculty member with clinical practice responsibilities, patient care service will be an important component of your role. Many pharmacists are attracted to positions as clinical faculty because these positions allow them to combine their desires for patient care and working with other health care professionals with the ability to teach and prepare the next generation of pharmacists for practice.

Patient care is especially appealing to clinical faculty members because, unlike faculty who teach in the classroom, they see the impact of their work relatively quickly. Clinical faculty not only care for patients and interact with other health care professionals but they also serve on committees within their health care facilities, such as the pharmacy and therapeutics committee, and they educate both students and other health care professionals.

Of course, patient care service needs to be balanced with other faculty commitments. Clinical faculty members must consult with their department chair and practice site supervisor to determine just how much time they should allocate to patient care and site service activities—teaching, scholarship, and service—outside their practice site.

Advancing the Profession

Pharmacy faculty play an important role in advancing the goals of their profession, usually through membership and service in professional organizations and societies. Many faculty members became active in service to their profession while they were still in school through groups such as the American Pharmacists Association (APhA) Academy of Student Pharmacists.

Service in professional organizations and societies benefits pharmacy faculty in many ways, including opportunities for:

- Education
- Professional development
- Leadership roles
- Serving as faculty advisors to students
- Advocating the organization's goals

Service to these groups—whether as an educator, health professional, or scientist—is essential for the continued development of our fields. Just as pharmacy faculty members have the responsibility to develop programs at their colleges, they also have the responsibility to shape the future of their disciplines.

Consulting

As pharmacists and scientists, pharmacy faculty possess specialized knowledge that can benefit many people outside of universities, patient care facilities, and professional organizations. A useful way to share this knowledge is through consulting.

For example, pharmacy faculty might serve as consultants to the pharmaceutical industry in a number of ways, such as the following.

- Clinical pharmacy faculty advise drug developers on the appropriate therapeutic uses of their products.
- Pharmaceutical sciences faculty work with the industry to develop and test new drugs and delivery methods.
- Economic, social, and administrative science faculty perform economic analyses of the outcomes of medication use (pharma-

coeconomics), develop marketing strategies for drug products, and assist with the legal and regulatory aspects of drug approval and use.

Pharmacy faculty members also have opportunities to consult for professional organizations, governmental agencies, not-for-profit organizations, book and journal publishers, and other professionals such as physicians, veterinarians, and attorneys.

Policies regarding the types of consulting activities that faculty can perform vary widely among colleges and universities. Some allow faculty to set time aside for consulting—often up to one day a week—and to keep the money earned through consulting activities. Others discourage consulting by limiting the amount of money faculty members can make outside of their university service, and some ban consulting entirely.

Also important to recognize is that many colleges and universities will not count a faculty member's consulting service as highly as their teaching, scholarship, or other types of service when it comes to preparing for promotion and tenure (see Chapters 3 and 7). You would be wise to consult your college and university policies and administrators before pursuing consulting opportunities.

Community Service

Many pharmacy faculty members gain a great deal of personal satisfaction by serving their communities. Opportunities to apply our specialized knowledge in community service include:

- Assisting patients at a free clinic.
- Conducting brown bag medication reviews.
- Presenting an educational seminar at a community or senior center.
- Helping Medicare-eligible patients select a Part D drug plan.
- Educating the public about aspects of medication use such as drug abuse, immunizations, or appropriate medication disposal.

Many faculty members volunteer for service activities that are not related to pharmacy, such as volunteering at their church, temple, or synagogue, serving food at a homeless shelter, or helping at an animal shelter. The community service provided by pharmacy faculty reflects well not only on themselves, but also on their programs, their schools and colleges, and our profession.

Documenting Your Activities

As a pharmacy faculty member you will be asked to document your teaching, scholarly activities, and service. Not only will this be important in tracking your progress as a faculty member, but also in developing a portfolio you will use to pursue promotion and tenure at your institution.

One way that faculty members track professional activities is by developing a curriculum vitae (CV). Unlike a résumé, which summarizes in one or two pages your qualifications for a particular position, a CV describes in greater detail all relevant activities you have been involved in over the course of your career. One of several resources available to help pharmacy faculty members prepare a CV is *The Pharmacy Professional's Guide to Résumés, CVs, & Interviewing* by Thomas P. Reinders, which is published by APhA.

Many colleges of pharmacy may ask you to develop an academic portfolio—which is a similar process to the one you followed to produce a portfolio as you progressed through school. Faculty members use portfolios to document their significant achievements in teaching, scholarship, and service and to make it easy for readers to track the progress they've made as a faculty member over time. Portfolios commonly include reflective narratives highlighting significant achievements and describing future goals in teaching, scholarship, and service. When faculty members are up for promotion or tenure they commonly create dossiers that also include these reflective narratives.

> Pharmacy faculty play an important role in advancing the goals of their profession, usually through membership and service in professional organizations and societies.

New pharmacy faculty members often struggle with how to classify activities on their CV or in their portfolios. For example, lecturing to a group of student pharmacists is commonly thought of as teaching, but it's less clear-cut if you are telling the students about a new discovery you made in your laboratory or at your practice site—which is an example of the teaching–research nexus mentioned on page 17.

What if you are experimenting with new methods of teaching to determine which results in better learning outcomes for your students? Or what if you are using your knowledge of a particular disease state to develop a new clinical service for your patients? The faculty at Midwestern University Chicago College of Pharmacy addressed the classification issue by integrating Boyer's scholarship paradigm with the academic triad. They developed the diagram shown in Figure 2-1 to help their faculty better understand and describe the multifaceted aspects of their work.

For example, when faculty members are preparing a scholarship narrative for a portfolio or promotion and tenure dossier, the diagram helps them realize that they should include not only examples of their research (Discovery of Knowledge), but also examples of how they:

- Put together existing facts to learn new knowledge (Integration and Organization of Knowledge).
- Used their knowledge to develop unique approaches to solving important problems (Application of Knowledge).
- Tested new methods of pedagogy to evaluate their effectiveness (Dissemination of Knowledge).

Figure 2-1 | Integrating Boyer's Four Areas of Scholarship into the Three Traditional Areas of Academic Performance

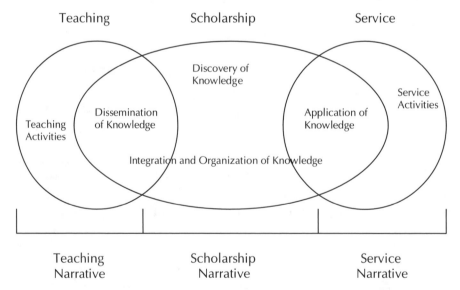

Source: *Midwestern University Chicago College of Pharmacy Faculty Handbook (internal document). Used with permission.*

Conclusion

You're likely beginning to realize that pharmacy faculty juggle many seemingly unrelated activities, yet integrate them in such a way that they come together into what can be an incredibly satisfying career path.

Getting the most out of a career as a pharmacy faculty member requires an understanding of not only teaching, scholarship, and service, but also of the environment where faculty members work. The next chapter will begin to describe the unique academic environment from the perspective of those who make a career in this setting.

Where to Find More Information on the Academic Triad

American Association of Colleges of Pharmacy (AACP)
Education Scholar Program
www.aacp.org/career/educationscholar/Pages/default.aspx
A program consisting of six online modules to expand the knowledge and skills of health professions educators. Includes a combination of on-screen text, images, and audio clips as well as examples, case studies, and demonstrations.

American College of Clinical Pharmacy (ACCP)
Academy Teaching and Learning Certificate Program
www.accp.com/academy/teachingAndLearning.aspx
A curriculum of live, interactive workshops offered by nationally known faculty and preceptors at ACCP's spring and fall meetings. Designed to prepare clinical pharmacy educators for didactic and experiential teaching. Awards a certificate of completion once the participant completes the program requirements.

American Journal of Pharmaceutical Education
www.ajpe.org
The official publication of the American Association of Colleges of Pharmacy. This peer-reviewed journal publishes original research, descriptions of innovations in teaching, articles about instructional design and assessment, and viewpoints pertaining to pharmacy education.

continued on page 24

continued from page 23

Currents in Pharmacy Teaching and Learning
www.elsevier.com/wps/find/journaldescription.cws_home/718643/
description
A peer-reviewed pharmacy education journal focusing on reports of in-novative teaching and learning strategies, skills development, outcomes assessment, curricular revision, and practical tips from seasoned educators.

The Pharmacy Professional's Guide to Résumés, CVs, & Interviewing, 2nd ed.
Reinders TP. Washington, DC: American Pharmacists Association; 2006
A book and CD-ROM with tips and examples to help pharmacists prepare cover letters, résumés, and curricula vitae and get ready for interviews.

Scholarship Reconsidered: Priorities of the Professoriate
Boyer EL. New York: Jossey-Bass; 1997
An important study completed by Ernest Boyer and the Carnegie Founda-tion for the Advancement of Teaching, presented in this ground-breaking book, resulted in a re-evaluation of how the work of faculty is assessed at many colleges and universities.

Chapter 3
Academia's Structure

"If you've seen one, you've seen them all" is a saying that, at first glance, you might think applies to the more than 110 pharmacy schools and colleges in the United States. After all, their missions are similar: to prepare students to become pharmacists, to carry out research and other forms of scholarship, and to serve patients, the profession, and the community. But in reality, each school and college has characteristics that make it unique.

How Colleges and Universities Are Organized

If you are a prospective or new pharmacy faculty member, you should make every effort to understand the workings of your college and university. Like anyone starting a new job, the more you know about your employer in advance, the better your chances of being successful in your position. Most likely your role will be a combination of teaching, scholarship, and service, as discussed in Chapter 2, but factors specific to your institution will affect how you perform these functions.

Similar to other large companies, colleges and universities employ large numbers of people who carry out a variety of functions. But working for an academic institution can be very different from working in other settings because the mission and structure of academia are unique.

For-Profit vs. Not-for-Profit

Practically all colleges and universities operate as not-for-profit organizations, meaning that their primary purpose is to provide services to their communities rather than a return on their stockholders' investments. Operating as not-for-profit organizations does not imply that the financial aspects of running a university are any less important or complicated than they are in for-profit companies.

All colleges and universities receive money from a variety of sources such as tuition, grants, donations, appropriations from state and federal governments, loans and lines of credit from banks, bonds, and sales of goods and services. And as with for-profit organizations, colleges and universities can't spend more than they bring in over the long term if they want to keep operating. They use the revenues that remain after expenses are paid to reinvest in their own institutions. (Note: What would be referred to as a *profit* in other businesses is commonly called a *fund balance* by not-for-profit organizations.)

Although colleges and universities typically don't have stockholders, they do have many constituencies with a vested interest in seeing the institution survive and thrive financially—including students and alumni, faculty and staff, governments, and the general public.

Public vs. Private

Understanding how colleges and universities work includes recognizing where funds come from to operate them and which people and groups influence a school's strategic planning and direction. A good first step is to identify whether your college or university is affiliated with some form of government, which means it is classified as a *public* university. Schools that are not affiliated with government are typically classified as *private*.

Public Universities

In general, a public university has a broad mission to serve the people affiliated with that level of government. Most public universities are affiliated with state governments, while a smaller number are affiliated with county and city governments or the federal government.

> Understanding a college of pharmacy's role and place within its university will help you better understand what may be expected of you as a faculty member as well as the resources available to help you do your job.

Traditionally, one of the primary missions of a public university is to provide educational opportunities to constituents who may not be able to afford an education at a private university. The government appropriates funds to the university and the university provides a tuition discount to residents. This arrangement benefits not only students by enabling them to receive an education at a lower cost, but also the government and its citizens by providing them with an educated workforce, including an adequate supply of health care workers and other professionals.

Public universities receive a government appropriation but they also rely on other forms of revenue, including tuition, grants, donations, funds from loans and bonds (which must be paid back), and sales of goods and services that can range from a surgical procedure at a university-owned medical center to a seat at a football or basketball game.

A challenge that many states and other governments face is how to continue financing the higher education needs of their citizens given competing demands and a limited amount of revenue, much of it generated through taxes. Many public universities have seen their appropriations fall short of their increases in expenses. The challenge for university administrators, and ultimately for programs such as colleges of pharmacy, is determining how to operate in an environment with fewer resources.

Private Universities

Private universities typically do not receive appropriations from governments; their students, however, are generally eligible for government-supported financial aid programs. Although private universities cannot rely on government revenue, they have the ability to determine their own missions and goals to best fit their unique needs. For example, many private universities in the United States are affiliated with religious groups. Often these schools have a mission to provide students an education within the context of the group's beliefs.

Similar to public universities, private universities must generate revenues from a variety of sources to cover the costs of their programs. A challenge faced by many private universities is sufficiently diversifying their sources of revenue. If a private university relies too much on a single source, such as tuition, donations, or endowment funds, it may be putting its programs, and even its own survival, at risk if something impacts that source.

Commonalities and Differences

From a student or faculty member's perspective, public and private universities have a number of characteristics in common. Both are involved in teaching, scholarship, and service. The degree of involvement can vary among institutions, however. For example, public universities—particularly those with colleges of pharmacy—often have larger enrollments and a larger number of majors and programs, and they are more likely to emphasize research as part of their mission as compared to private universities.

Although private universities often have smaller enrollments and missions that focus more on teaching, don't assume that this will always be the case. Some private universities are very large and have research-intensive missions. And some public universities are relatively small, often with a mission focused on one particular area.

Where Colleges of Pharmacy Fit

How do colleges of pharmacy fit into the organizational structure described above? Although this may sound like a simple question, it by no means has a simple answer.

Colleges of pharmacy are found within both public and private universities. They are found within large, research-intensive universities as well as smaller, teaching-intensive institutions. In some cases a college of pharmacy may stand alone as a single program on which a university is based, or be part of a small group of programs all related to a similar discipline, such as a university whose mission focuses on the health sciences.

Understanding a college of pharmacy's role and place within its university will help you better understand what may be expected of you as a faculty member as well as the resources available to help you do your job. Key factors to consider regarding the college of pharmacy's placement, summarized in Table 3-1, are discussed in more detail below.

Large vs. Small Institutions

Advantages of working at a pharmacy college within a large university include access to a vast pool of university resources, from research equipment and specially trained personnel to centers dedicated to helping faculty with technology or teaching. These colleges tend to be relatively small units in a much larger university, which creates a sense of camaraderie among the faculty, staff, and students. Thus you get the combined advantages of a small college "feel" along with access to the resources of a large university.

However, large universities can be administratively complex, making it difficult to find and get hold of services when you need them. And the goals, objectives, and resource needs of a college of pharmacy may be different from those of the larger university, particularly if few other programs on your campus train health professionals.

On the other hand, some colleges of pharmacy may be central to, or a significant part of, the university's mission, especially if the university is smaller or highly mission-focused. The college of pharmacy's goals, objectives, and resource needs may constitute a significant component of the needs of the entire institution, boosting chances that the college's voice will be heard. In these

Table 3-1 | Factors to Consider Regarding College of Pharmacy Settings

	Pros	Cons
In Large Universities	• Access to a large pool of university resources including research equipment, personnel, and centers to help faculty with technology or teaching. • Strong sense of camaraderie and small-college feel.	• Administratively complex, making it difficult to access services when you need them. • College of pharmacy goals, objectives, and resource needs may differ from those of the larger university.
In Small Universities	• College of pharmacy and university goals may be highly aligned, giving the college a strong voice. • Students and faculty may form relationships more easily across the university's disciplines.	• Fewer resources to draw from. • Small, collegial atmosphere may seem too political or intrusive to some faculty.
In Academic Medical Centers	• Rewarding for college of pharmacy faculty who want to teach, conduct research, and practice with health professionals and researchers across health disciplines.	• Limitations on access to resources. • Fewer opportunities to interact with colleagues and students outside of health care.

smaller universities, resources can be easier to access and the atmosphere may be one in which students and faculty form relationships not only within their programs, but across the university's disciplines.

Disadvantages to working at smaller colleges of pharmacy at smaller universities generally include fewer resources on which to draw, especially if the college is not related to the university's mission. For example, a pharmacy faculty member who used to be part of a larger university and collaborated with faculty from the business school or an education program may find such colleagues absent at a smaller school. The collegial atmosphere at a pharmacy school in a small university, which some faculty find so attractive, may actually drive others away, particularly those who want to "avoid campus politics" or "focus on my work without unrelated interruptions."

Academic Medical Centers

Some colleges of pharmacy are affiliated with academic medical centers, which usually consist of large hospitals and networks of health providers whose missions are related to teaching, scholarship, and patient care. Academic medical centers are part of or directly affiliated with colleges of medicine, pharmacy, nursing, or other health professions.

Working at an academic medical center can be especially rewarding for college of pharmacy faculty who desire to teach, conduct research, and practice with other health professionals and researchers across health disciplines. Affiliation with an academic medical center provides a sense of institutional mission and purpose that is consistent with the reason many people select health care careers in the first place.

> Working at an academic medical center can be especially rewarding for college of pharmacy faculty who desire to teach, conduct research, and practice with other health professionals and researchers across health disciplines.

Disadvantages of being part of an academic medical center are similar to those associated with smaller universities, especially regarding limited access to resources. For those who want to interact with colleagues and students outside of health care, an academic medical center might be a professionally stifling environment.

Established vs. New Programs

With the rapid growth in the number of colleges of pharmacy—from fewer than 80 in 1990 to nearly 120 today (as shown in Figure 1-1)—you are likely to have choices between working at a long-established college of pharmacy or taking a position in a relatively new program. Joining a newer pharmacy school can be exciting, whether it's your first position or you're an experienced pharmacy educator, because you're poised to shape practically everything about your program, including curriculum structure, teaching methods, student selection, research initiatives, faculty recruitment, promotion, and tenure policies. You'll likely form powerful bonds with students and colleagues as you work together to create a program, resulting in a strong sense of camaraderie.

Some of the most exciting aspects of being part of a new program can also be the most challenging. Not having a history of how things were done in the past can lead you in thrilling new directions, but it also means that you may not have the experience to recognize potential problems and how to best deal with them.

Faculty members at new pharmacy schools often spend a great deal of time on the teaching and service activities necessary to establish their programs—in many cases, at the expense of scholarly productivity. It's important to understand how this allocation of effort will be viewed in the context of workload planning, promotion, and tenure. Will colleagues and administrators at your university recognize the valid reasons why your productivity may differ from that of others in your field at more established institutions? Will peers at other institutions recognize the unique work you carried out to help establish your program and how it may have impacted your productivity? These are questions you will want to ask during the employment search and interview processes (see Chapter 5).

Administrative Structure of Colleges of Pharmacy

When you're new to any organization you need to take steps to learn the administrative structure and chain of command. This not only helps you understand who reports to whom and how things get done, but it also introduces you to the intricacies of the human and political relationships inherent in the organization so you can function effectively.

The Leadership Team

Most pharmacy schools have a similar administrative structure and leadership team, described in the following sections. Table 3-2 summarizes this information.

The Dean

The central authority for all colleges of pharmacy, the dean is formally the college's chief academic and administrative officer. The dean also holds important leadership roles within his or her college, university, and profession.

Deans have distinguished themselves throughout their careers, typically by earning solid credentials as teachers and scholars at universities, but occasionally they stand out because of their experience and leadership in corporations and other organizations. Deans need the leadership skills to inspire the college's faculty, staff, and students along with the managerial skills to operate a large, complex organization within an organization. Although the dean is ultimately responsible for all aspects of the college of pharmacy, he or she must

Table 3-2 | Key Administrative Roles in Colleges of Pharmacy

	Responsibilities	Typical Qualifications
The College Dean	• The college's chief academic and administrative officer. • Holds important leadership roles within the college, university, and profession. • Typically reports to a provost or other university administrator. • Interacts with the university chief executive officer, especially regarding the university's mission or fundraising. • Serves as official spokesperson and represents the college's interests to other groups. • Helps obtain resources from agencies, donors, and others.	• Has led a distinguished career. • A doctoral-level degree (usually a PhD or a PharmD). • Typically has solid credentials as teacher and scholar; may have experience in corporations and other organizations. • Possesses leadership skills to inspire faculty, staff, and students. • Has managerial skills to operate a large, complex organization.
Other Deans	• Support the dean regarding operational areas such as student affairs, professional affairs, academic affairs, clinical and professional education, etc. • Common titles are associate or assistant dean.	• Often are experienced faculty members with expertise in a particular operating area, such as professional affairs, clinical education, or assessment. • Some have expertise outside of academia or clinical practice, such as administration and operations, student affairs, or development.

continued on page 33

Table 3-2 | *continued from page 32*

	Responsibilities	**Typical Qualifications**
Chairs	• Head the pharmacy college's academic units (usually departments or divisions). • Report directly to the dean and oversee day-to-day operations of the department. • Common departments in pharmacy schools are pharmaceutical sciences and pharmacy practice. • Other departments may include pharmacology, pharmaceutics, medicinal chemistry, social and administrative sciences, clinical and experimental therapeutics, and clinical pharmacy practice. • Oversee administrative tasks such as course scheduling, hiring, evaluations, and budget. • Mentor and assist faculty with day-to-day issues.	• Experienced faculty members who excel in their area of expertise. • History of leadership, particularly in guiding faculty to develop strategic plans and goals for their units.
Directors	• Lead program related to the college's mission, such as research centers, graduate programs, residency programs, and research fellowships.	• Often are faculty members or researchers with experience in the area pertaining to the center they direct.

delegate many administrative and leadership functions to be sure that they are performed efficiently and effectively.

The dean serves as the college of pharmacy's official spokesperson and represents the college's interests to constituencies within the university, such as other college deans, university administrators, and the board of trustees, as well as to all external groups, including the state and national associations representing the pharmacy profession. In addition to heading the college of pharmacy, the dean typically reports to other administrators within the university, such as a provost, who is the chief academic officer at most universities, or to a vice president for academic affairs, who is the chief education officer within an academic medical center. Deans commonly interact with the chief executive officer of the university—often a president or chancellor—especially with regard to helping to shape the university's mission or fundraising.

The dean is also called on to help obtain resources for the college from a variety of sources, including university administrators, governmental agencies, alumni, and other potential donors.

New pharmacy faculty members are not likely to report directly to the dean, even though the dean may have made the final decision regarding offering you a position. However, the dean will play a very important role in shaping the environment at your college, especially regarding your program's mission and vision, policies and procedures, and relationships with external constituencies such as medical centers, clinics, and pharmacies. The outcomes of your dean's work are likely to impact your activities as a faculty member on a daily basis.

Other College Administrators
The structure of each college of pharmacy's reporting relationships varies. In most cases the dean is supported by other college administrators, including associate or assistant deans who are typically responsible for important operational aspects of the college, such as student affairs, professional affairs, academic affairs, clinical and professional education, assessment, research, graduate and postgraduate programs, alumni relations and development, etc. These administrators tend to be experienced faculty members or professional staff with extensive experience in the areas for which they are responsible.

The academic units of a college of pharmacy, usually called departments or divisions, typically have chairs who report directly to the dean and are members of the college's administrative team. These department chairs tend to be experienced faculty members who have distinguished themselves by their teaching, scholarship, and service within their areas of expertise.

Deans are also supported by professional staff such as administrative assistants, admissions officers, facilities managers, and advancement and development personnel who perform such essential functions as creating academic and course calendars and keeping the college's facilities functioning and secure.

Colleges and universities commonly operate programs related to their missions, such as research centers, graduate programs, residency programs, and research fellowships. Each is led by a director—usually a faculty member in the college with expertise in the program or center—who reports to the dean or another administrator. Pharmacy faculty members often work with these centers and programs in addition to handling their responsibilities at the college.

The Department Chair

When you're getting started as a pharmacy faculty member, your primary contact with the college's administrative team will likely be through the department chair. A department chair is an administrator in charge of an academic unit within a college.

Most colleges of pharmacy have at least two academic departments or divisions: pharmaceutical sciences and pharmacy practice. Some colleges have more than two, particularly those with larger numbers of faculty across a variety of specialty areas, such as pharmacology, pharmaceutics, medicinal chemistry, social and administrative sciences, clinical and experimental therapeutics, and clinical pharmacy practice. During your pre-employment research or interview, clarify to which department you will be assigned. For example, at some colleges of pharmacy, social and administrative scientists are part of the pharmaceutical sciences department, at others they are part of pharmacy practice, and at some colleges they have their own department.

Department chairs tend to be experienced faculty members who have distinguished themselves within their area of expertise. They report directly to the dean and are responsible for leading the faculty and overseeing day-to-day operations of the department.

Joining a newer pharmacy school can be exciting, whether it's your first position or you're an experienced pharmacy educator, because you're positioned to shape nearly everything, including curriculum structure, teaching methods, student selection, research initiatives, faculty recruitment, promotion, and tenure policies.

Duties of the chair include administrative tasks such as seeing that courses get scheduled, hiring faculty and staff, developing and evaluating faculty, and overseeing the department's budget. Department chairs are expected to display leadership, particularly in guiding their faculty to develop strategic plans and goals for their units. They are also responsible for working with individual faculty members on activities ranging from assigning teaching and service workloads to serving as a sounding board on day-to-day issues and mentoring faculty to help them achieve their short- and long-term career goals.

Because your department chair will likely be your direct supervisor, you should develop a solid relationship with him or her early in your career. Even better, develop this relationship before you begin your position! Your chair can play a vital role in helping you navigate your way through the college and university and can connect you with resources to help you develop the quality of your teaching, scholarship, and service activities. As an experienced faculty member, your chair will likely have a good feel for the issues you will face early in your career and can help you manage these issues by sharing his or her own experiences, connecting you with others who can help, or simply being someone who will listen.

Although department chairs can provide guidance and resources, it is up to you as a faculty member to perform at the level expected by your department, college, and university. In other words, you are ultimately responsible for your own success in academia. Besides understanding what your department chair can do for you, recognize what he or she can't do. Department chairs are classic examples of "middle management" within large organizations—possessing the resources to help with some issues but needing to consult others in the organization before they can take action. For example, a department chair may need permission from the dean or provost before he or she can adjust your workload to allow you to pursue a special project.

Faculty Appointments

When you start your career as a new pharmacy faculty member you'll receive an "academic appointment" to a particular rank that is consistent with your experience and achievements. These ranks are summarized in Table 3-3.

Qualifications for an entry-level rank as well as for promotion to higher ranks can vary considerably among institutions, so consult your university's faculty bylaws and policies and procedures (commonly referred to as the faculty hand-

Table 3-3 | **Key Faculty Roles in Colleges of Pharmacy**

Lecturer or Instructor	• Faculty with little or no experience and no terminal degree (PharmD or PhD) in their field. • Help teach courses with laboratories or discussion sections.
Adjunct Instructor	• Instructor who teaches for but is not employed by the university. • Often is a volunteer preceptor of introductory and advanced pharmacy practice experiences.
Assistant Professor	• Has a terminal degree (PharmD, PhD) and some teaching and research experience. • Shows promise for future professional growth.
Associate Professor	• Teaching, scholarship, and service records surpass expectations for entry-level faculty. • Is developing a reputation with peers at other institutions. • Shows promise for continued professional growth.
Professor	• Highest rank assigned by academic institutions. • Has a record of outstanding teaching, scholarship, and service. • Often has a national or international reputation in a specific field.

book) and check with your dean and department chair to learn the promotion expectations within your department, college, and university.

Lecturer or Instructor

Appointments given to faculty members who have little or no experience, or who have not completed a terminal degree in their field (PharmD, PhD), are typically as a lecturer or an instructor. Faculty members in these positions often help teach courses with laboratories or lead discussion sections.

Adjunct Instructor

Adjunct instructors are those who teach for, but are not employed by, the university. At pharmacy schools, the title of adjunct instructor is typically given to preceptors of introductory and advanced pharmacy practice experiences.

Assistant Professor

Most new faculty members will enter the academic ranks as an assistant professor. The assistant professor rank is commonly given to faculty members who have obtained their terminal degree and have also garnered enough experience to qualify them to begin a career in academia.

In colleges of pharmacy, assistant professors in pharmacy practice departments commonly have a doctor of pharmacy (PharmD) degree and have completed post-doctoral residency or fellowship training. Assistant professors in social and administrative sciences or pharmaceutical sciences typically have a doctor of philosophy (PhD) degree and have obtained additional teaching and research experience, often as a teaching assistant or by completing postdoctoral research work.

Associate Professor

To earn the rank of associate professor, you must perform beyond the expectations of an entry-level faculty member and show promise for future professional growth. Typically, associate professorship is conferred to assistant professors who, as demonstrated through their records of teaching, scholarship, and service, have met or surpassed the expectations set by their institutions.

New pharmacy faculty members may occasionally start at this rank, especially if they have a record of professional achievements and experience similar to other associate professors at the hiring institution. The expectations for promotion, as well as the ability to start at a rank higher than assistant professor, vary widely between institutions. Learning about the expectations for initial rank and promotion to higher ranks should be part of your employment assessment process (see Chapter 5).

Professor

The highest rank assigned by academic institutions is professor. Faculty obtaining this rank must have long and distinguished records of teaching, scholarship, and service. Many institutions also require professors to have built national or international reputations within their fields and be recognized for leadership in their institutions and professions.

Most institutions require that faculty members spend time as assistant and associate professors and meet internal standards for achievements in teaching, scholarship, and service before they can apply to become professors. Although some institutions may hire a new faculty member directly into the rank of professor, this practice is exceptionally rare because people outside of academia have very few opportunities to develop a strong record of teaching, scholarship, and service.

Appointment Terms

Your faculty appointment may be described as academic year or calendar year, and tenure track or non-tenure track.

Academic Year

Academic-year appointments typically require faculty to work for the university during the regular eight- or nine-month school term, usually starting with the beginning of the fall session and ending at the conclusion of spring session. Faculty members on these appointments are not expected to work for the university when the students are off, such as during breaks between sessions and during the summer. Often faculty use the three or four months away from their duties to work on scholarship activities or enhance their professional development. In many cases they seek funding from external sources to supplement their salaries during this time.

Academic-year appointments were very common in the past, but increasingly universities—and especially colleges of pharmacy—expect faculty to carry out teaching, scholarship, and service activities throughout the year. Some faculty on academic-year appointments value the time away from the classroom, while others are conflicted by the demands of having to fulfill 12 months' worth of job expectations while being paid less than if they had a calendar-year appointment.

Calendar Year

Faculty on calendar-year appointments are expected to work for their universities all year long. Rather than taking breaks when students are away, these faculty, like employees at most other kinds of organizations, get paid based on an expectation of being at work every day, and they commonly receive paid-time-off benefits such as vacation and professional leave.

Calendar-year appointments recognize that teaching, scholarship, and service—especially patient-care activities—take place throughout the year. According to 2009 data from the American Association of Colleges of Pharmacy, 87% of full-time faculty members are now on calendar-year appointments.

Tenure Track

Faculty members on tenure-track appointments are initially offered probationary contracts, which means that their performance is evaluated regularly based on their institution's expectations for teaching, scholarship, and service. Near the end of the probationary period, which typically lasts five to six years, you submit a portfolio of your work (often referred to as a *dossier*) that is reviewed extensively by faculty colleagues in your institution and by external peers in your professional field. If you are judged to meet your institution's performance standards you are offered tenure, which takes you off probationary status and usually extends to you a new contract without an explicit term.

Faculty who achieve tenure can often remain at their institutions until they voluntarily choose to leave, as long as they continue to meet institutional performance standards. At some institutions these standards are minimal, such as requiring that you not be found incompetent or engaging in immoral actions, while at others, there is a post-tenure review process in which the quality of your teaching, scholarship, and service continue to be evaluated.

Those on the tenure track often find the process of obtaining tenure stressful, but achieving tenure provides opportunities you rarely find in any other line of work. This "lifetime contract" gives tenured faculty a great deal of leeway to pursue their own teaching, scholarly, and service interests.

> Faculty who achieve tenure can often remain at their institutions until they voluntarily choose to leave, as long as they continue to meet institutional performance standards.

Non-tenure Track

If you're on a non-tenure-track appointment your contract has a finite term, typically one to three years at most institutions. Decisions regarding reappointment are generally based on whether you've met performance expectations, but they can also be influenced by other factors. For example, a contract may not be renewed if a college makes a curricular change in which a course taught by a non-tenure-track faculty member is no longer part of the program. Although non-tenure-track faculty members are not able to obtain tenure, most are eligible for promotion.

Criteria for promotion vary among institutions and also between non-tenure-track and tenure-track faculty. Those not on the tenure track are often evaluated with greater emphasis on only one or two components of the academic triad (usually teaching and service), while tenure-track faculty are usually evaluated on all three components—the weight of each mirroring what's emphasized in the institution's mission and goals.

Clinical Track

At most institutions, clinical-track contracts are essentially non-tenure-track contracts that pertain to the distinct job responsibilities of clinical practitioners who care for patients while also performing traditional faculty functions. Since these faculty members focus primarily on clinical practice, it would be difficult to judge them on the same teaching, scholarship, and service expectations that campus-based faculty are measured by.

Clinical-track faculty commonly hold joint appointments with both a university and their clinical practice site, such as a hospital, clinic, or pharmacy. Appointments with the university tend to be for a finite term (usually one year), and may or may not be related to the faculty member's contract with their clinical sites. For example, if the partnership between a college of pharmacy and a clinical site changes, a pharmacist's clinical faculty appointment may not be renewed but his or her status as a practitioner at the site will remain unaffected.

A clinical track faculty member's job responsibilities may vary based on the source of funding for the position. The money to fund a clinical track faculty position may come entirely from the college of pharmacy, entirely from the clinical practice site, or from a combination of the two groups. Clinical track faculty often feel that they have two "bosses"—one at the college of pharmacy and one at their practice site.

Knowing the funding arrangements for your position may simplify some matters, while complicating others. You may be asked to take on more responsibilities at the site that provides your funding; at the same time, you're likely to feel you are missing out on important activities at the other site when you're not there. Good communication between the college, practice site, and faculty member is essential to managing the ambiguities and pressures of having responsibilities at more than one place.

How Colleges of Pharmacy Obtain Financial Resources

Your specific roles and responsibilities as a faculty member at a college of pharmacy are likely to be affected by how your college obtains the resources it needs to operate. As part of an organization within an organization, administrators at pharmacy colleges often work with university administrators to procure resources necessary for the college's day-to-day operations. For example, the dean of the college of pharmacy may negotiate with university administrators for funds to hire faculty and staff, acquire space on campus for faculty to teach and perform research, and pay for overhead expenses—everything from computers and laboratory equipment to copy machines and paper clips.

Whether your college of pharmacy is part of a public or private university, the dean and administrators must work to obtain external support if the college is to achieve its mission and goals, such as educating more students, performing new types of research, and developing new teaching methods. The university's internal resources are limited; when college of pharmacy administrators make a case for additional support, they are competing with other colleges and programs that are also seeking support for their missions.

Among the many sources that colleges of pharmacy can look to for external funding are alumni and friends of the college, government agencies, charitable foundations, and corporations—especially those likely to employ the college's graduates or benefit from their research and service activities. The size of these external gifts can be as small as a few dollars for a pharmacy student activity or as large as several million dollars donated to support an endowed professorship or the construction of a new building.

Helping to Obtain Funds

You may be wondering what impact these financial matters have on your work as a pharmacy faculty member. Although funds obtained by college and university administrators may support much of your work, you might be asked to obtain additional resources to cover some of your activities. Faculty members who conduct research and scholarship activities are commonly required to seek grants and other funding to support their work. Obtaining funding is especially important for tenure-track faculty required to produce peer-reviewed publications and presentations based on their research.

Shared Appointments

Colleges of pharmacy often reach out to other entities inside and outside their institutions to share costs, giving all parties access to resources they could not obtain on their own, such as teaching and research facilities, libraries and learning resources, and personnel.

For example, a college of pharmacy may work with another program to offer a faculty member a joint appointment, such as a pharmacology professor having joint appointments in the colleges of pharmacy and medicine. Colleges of pharmacy also join up with pharmacies, hospitals, clinics, and other health facilities to support pharmacists who have practice responsibilities at their clinical site and academic responsibilities at the college. Such arrangements are commonly referred to as cofunded or shared appointments.

If you are considering a joint, cofunded, or shared appointment, there are several important factors to consider, such as determining which party involved in the appointment will be your "home" and responsible for assigning your workload and setting your performance expectations. Even though a pharmacy school and a hospital may agree to equally share the costs of a cofunded faculty member, and the faculty member spends most of his time at the hospital doing patient care and teaching, the college of pharmacy may assign his workload and evaluate him. All parties (college of pharmacy, cofunding partner, the faculty member, and other personnel at the college and partner site) must come to a clear understanding of these vital issues to avoid confusion and stress for the faculty member and partners.

Conclusion

This chapter introduced you to how colleges and universities are structured— general information helpful to know before taking a position as a pharmacy faculty member, but by no means all-inclusive.

Every university and college of pharmacy is unique. Certain things are impossible to learn about your institution until you start your career and get first-hand experience. Give yourself time to learn your institution's intricacies and the expectations others have of you as a faculty member.

Experienced faculty members often say it takes at least a full year, and often longer, to get a feel for all the issues related to your college's or university's op- erations. One thing most faculty members have in common is an appreciation for learning. You're apt to find that your colleagues are supportive and patient as you learn to become a pharmacy faculty member.

Where to Find More Information on Structure and Operations in Academia

American Association of Colleges of Pharmacy Annual Profile of Faculty
www.aacp.org/CAREER/SALARYDATA/Pages/default.aspx
An annual description of the demographics and salary information for college of pharmacy faculty members.

continued on page 44

continued from page 43

The Chronicle of Higher Education
www.chronicle.com
A newspaper and website dedicated to reporting on general issues
impacting university faculty and higher education.

Mentor in a Manual: Climbing the Academic Ladder to Tenure, 3rd ed.
Schoenfeld AC, Magnan R. Madison, Wis: Atwood Publications; 2004
A commonly referenced guide to the roles of teaching, scholarship, and
service at various stages of the tenure-track process.

**Handbook for Pharmacy Educators: Getting Adjusted as a
New Pharmacy Faculty Member**
Desselle SP, Hammer DP. Binghamton, NY: The Haworth Press; 2002
Personal accounts from junior faculty members at colleges of pharmacy
of their trials and tribulations on the path to promotion and tenure.

Currents in Pharmacy Teaching and Learning
Bruce SP, guest ed. August 2009;1(1):1-64
Launched in 2009 and published by Elsevier, the first issue of this journal
is dedicated to new clinical faculty development. Topics covered include
assessing your work style, how to evaluate positions in academia, and
balancing work and home life.

Chapter 4

Preparing for an Academic Career

One of the best aspects of the pharmacy profession is the variety of career paths you can follow. According to the American Pharmacists Association's Career Pathway Evaluation Program for Pharmacy Professionals, pharmacy has more than 25 specialty areas and many more subspecialties. Likewise, pharmacy faculty can follow many scientific, clinical, academic, and administrative career paths.

As with all journeys, you must start with a first step. If you are serious about launching a career as a pharmacy faculty member, you can prepare yourself in many ways.

Start Preparing in Pharmacy School

You can begin to get ready for an academic career while still in pharmacy school. Even though the doctor of pharmacy curriculum prepares graduates to be generalist practitioners, you can take steps now to build the specialized knowledge and experiences that faculty members need to enter academia.

The classroom, the laboratory, or a practice site is a great place to start. If you particularly enjoyed a certain subject or course, or if you found a clinical experience on a rotation especially interesting, then use this as a springboard to learn more about what it takes to specialize or gain added expertise in this area. Most pharmacy faculty members are hired not based on their abilities as a generalist, but on the degree of expertise they have gained in a particular area of practice or research.

As a student pharmacist, you are likely to have many opportunities to take elective courses, participate in introductory and advanced pharmacy practice experiences (IPPEs and APPEs), and work with faculty to learn more about particular topics and the degree of expertise necessary to become a pharmacy faculty member.

Colleges play an important role in developing the next generation of pharmacy faculty members. Some colleges offer courses specific to teaching methods and learning in which students become acquainted with pedagogical techniques useful in the classroom, laboratory, or practice site. Many colleges also offer APPEs in teaching and research that let students work alongside faculty to learn about teaching methods, course delivery, or the research process. Some schools also give student pharmacists employment opportunities as teaching or research assistants. All these options help you gain first-hand experience and assess whether a career as a pharmacy faculty member is something you wish to pursue further.

Experiences at the undergraduate and professional level are helpful, but most faculty positions in colleges of pharmacy require postgraduate training, which usually comes in the forms listed below:

- Residencies
- Fellowships
- Graduate study

The training you pursue should be driven by the skills you wish to acquire and the type of faculty position in which you are interested. This chapter provides details about various options. Table 4-1 offers a quick summary.

Residency Training

Residency training helps you advance your clinical practice skills. The primary purpose of residency training is to apply the knowledge and skills obtained in pharmacy school to "real world" experiences, such as caring for patients and managing a pharmacy practice.

> Some colleges offer courses specific to teaching methods and learning in which students become acquainted with pedagogical techniques useful in the classroom, laboratory, or practice site.

Residency training programs are structured to offer pharmacists many opportunities to gain a variety of experiences in a relatively short period (usually one or two years). Residents work closely with preceptors to continue the learning process they started in pharmacy school. In residencies the learning process is centered on clinical practice, often focusing on a particular setting (e.g., hospitals, ambulatory care clinics, managed care, community pharmacies) or a particular clinical specialty (e.g., infectious disease, cardiology, pediatrics). Residents are generally given more time to develop a new clinical

Table 4-1 | Postgraduate Training Options for Preparing to be a Pharmacy Faculty Member

	Residency Training	Fellowship Training	Graduate Study
Description	Introductory and advanced programs that allow pharmacists to develop clinical skills in real-world settings over one or two years.	Prepares you for a career as an independent clinical investigator by working closely with clinical researchers. Provides hands-on research experience over two or more years to gain skills necessary for carrying out clinical research projects.	Advanced academic work beyond a bachelor's or first professional degree; can be carried out in practically any discipline. Master's degrees typically take one to two years; doctoral degrees can take four or more years.
How it promotes your ability to become a faculty member	A common requirement for clinical faculty positions at colleges of pharmacy; often you need to complete both a PGY1 and a PGY2 residency. Try to seek programs in which you develop both your teaching and practice skills.	Prepares you for faculty positions with a clinical research component.	PhD required for most faculty positions in the pharmaceutical and social and administrative sciences; may also be required for pharmacy practice positions with a high research component. In some instances, postdoctoral research work is necessary before obtaining a faculty position.

service and evaluate practice models than they'd be given if they'd taken an entry-level staff pharmacist position immediately after leaving pharmacy school. Keep in mind that as a resident you are practicing as a pharmacist, so you will be given more independent responsibility for patient care and projects than you were as a student pharmacist.

Many pharmacists who complete residency programs report that the experience gave their careers a three- to five-year head start and believe the career opportunities open to them, including those in academia, would not have been otherwise available.

Residency Types

Residencies allow you to learn from experienced practitioners in a variety of settings, including hospitals, clinics, community pharmacies, and managed care organizations.

Many residencies are classified as postgraduate year 1 (PGY1) programs that emphasize the development of skills needed by "generalist" practitioners in a particular practice setting. Postgraduate year 2 (PGY2) programs usually provide advanced training in focused areas, such as clinical specialties or pharmacy practice management.

Residency training programs are accredited to assure consistency and quality across programs. Most residency programs are accredited by the American Society of Health-System Pharmacists (ASHP). ASHP works in partnership with the American Pharmacists Association (APhA) and the Academy of Managed Care Pharmacy (AMCP) to develop accreditation standards for community pharmacy and managed care residencies, respectively. Follow the links at the end of this chapter to learn more about residency training programs.

Completing a residency is a common requirement for clinical faculty positions at colleges of pharmacy. While some clinical faculty positions are available after completing a PGY1 residency, many call for specialization in a particular clinical area and experience with a particular practice setting. Gaining this level of specialization and experience may require completing both a PGY1 and a PGY2 residency.

Projects

All residency programs require trainees to complete a project, which helps you prepare for the types of scholarly activities expected of clinical faculty members. These projects, typically presented at regional and national conferences and occasionally published in peer-reviewed literature, tend to fall into two areas:

- Developing a new clinical service. An example would be implementing a travel medication clinic in a community pharmacy.
- Evaluating an existing clinical service. An example would be evaluating a clinical pharmacy hyperlipidemia service in a private physician's office.

Teaching

Residency programs, especially those associated with colleges of pharmacy, are increasingly integrating teaching and learning experiences into their training requirements. Residents in these programs have opportunities to lecture, facilitate laboratories and discussion sections, and precept student pharmacists on IPPEs and APPEs. They can also participate in seminars that specifically focus on developing teaching skills. Residents in these programs are often awarded a certificate signifying their additional training and experience in education.

People who have completed residencies that included teaching preparation are highly sought after to teach at colleges of pharmacy. If you are embarking on residency training with the intention of pursuing a clinical faculty position, make it a point to seek programs that offer opportunities to develop your teaching skills in addition to your pharmacy practice skills.

> The primary purpose of residency training is to apply the knowledge and skills obtained in pharmacy school to "real world" experiences, such as caring for patients and managing a pharmacy practice.

Fellowship Training

Unlike residency training, which focuses on developing clinical practice skills, a fellowship is a postgraduate training program that prepares you for a career as an independent clinical investigator.

Pharmacists in fellowship programs work closely with researchers and other investigators in a highly individualized program to learn the skills necessary to carry out a research project. Fellows often learn these skills through a combination of graduate-level coursework and hands-on research experience.

Fellowship programs are typically based in colleges of pharmacy or medicine, academic medical centers, the pharmaceutical industry, or specialized care institutions. Although the length of a fellowship follows no set timeline, most programs take two or more years to complete, which allows you to not only learn research skills, but also gain experience in writing grant proposals and research reports, as well as in preparing poster and podium presentations.

Most fellows leave their programs having helped to write research protocols, grants, and publications. Given these skills and experiences, pharmacists who complete a fellowship are prepared to enter faculty positions in which there is a significant expectation to conduct research in addition to teaching and service.

Because fellowship training is so individualized, no formal accreditation group exists for fellowship programs in pharmacy. However, the American College of Clinical Pharmacy (ACCP) has developed a document called *Guidelines for Clinical Research Fellowship Training Programs* that provides clear direction, such as training program requirements, preceptor qualifications, applicant criteria, and fellowship experiences. A number of fellowship programs participate in a voluntary peer review process administered by ACCP to ensure the quality of these programs. ACCP also provides a directory of pharmacy fellowship training programs.

> In fellowship programs, typically based in colleges of pharmacy or medicine, academic medical centers, the pharmaceutical industry, or specialized care institutions, you learn research skills and gain experience in writing grant proposals and research reports, as well as in preparing poster and podium presentations.

Graduate Study

Graduate study is advanced academic work beyond a bachelor's or first professional degree. Residencies and fellowships are inherently clinical in nature, but graduate studies can be carried out in practically any discipline, such as chemistry or biology, as well as between disciplines, such as pharmaceutics, which combines aspects of chemistry, biology, and pharmacy.

Graduate programs typically award either a master's degree, such as a master of science (MS), master of arts (MA), master of business administration (MBA), or master of public health (MPH). At a more advanced level you can earn a doctoral-level degree, such as a doctor of philosophy (PhD) or doctor of public health (DrPH).

Master's Degrees

Master's-level degrees place a heavy emphasis on coursework to help you build the knowledge inherent in a particular discipline or field, with an emphasis on how that information is applied. For example, students in MBA programs develop knowledge and skills that are important in business settings, especially for operating or administering an organization.

Master's degrees are generally designed to be wrapped up in about two years of full-time study, although many programs offer part-time options. Some master's programs will require you to complete a project or research thesis in addition to coursework.

Doctoral Degrees

Doctoral-level degrees usually combine the coursework and knowledge set in master's-level programs with additional coursework and research training to shape you into an investigator who can lead research studies independently.

Doctoral degrees usually take four or more years to complete because they combine a rigorous program of building knowledge and developing research skills. You almost always have to complete a capstone research project, commonly referred to as a dissertation, which shows that you have developed the skills necessary to function as an independent researcher.

Many Disciplines

As of 2010, 70 colleges of pharmacy offered graduate degree programs, which are available for virtually every discipline in the profession, such as:

- Pharmaceutical sciences
  - Pharmacology
  - Medicinal chemistry
  - Pharmaceutics

- Social and administrative sciences in pharmacy
  - Pharmacy management
  - Communications
  - Health care policy

- Clinical sciences
  - Clinical therapeutics
  - Experimental therapeutics

You can also take part in programs that cross disciplines, such as:

- Pharmacoeconomics—combining aspects of the social and administrative sciences with clinical pharmacy practice
- Nuclear pharmacy—combining clinical practice with pharmaceutics and physical chemistry

The disciplines bulleted on the previous page are just a sampling of programs available. For a full listing of the areas of study in master's and doctoral programs in U.S. colleges of pharmacy, see the link in the American Association of Colleges of Pharmacy (AACP) entry in the "For More Information" section at the end of this chapter. Graduate degree programs at colleges of pharmacy, unlike PharmD programs, are not subject to accreditation review.

Although some graduate programs require a professional degree in pharmacy, many admit students from other disciplines as long as their undergraduate training prepared them to be successful in graduate school. For example, many students in medicinal chemistry graduate programs have undergraduate degrees in chemistry and other sciences, and not in pharmacy.

Common Requirements

Colleges of pharmacy commonly require a graduate degree for faculty positions that focus more on research and teaching than on clinical practice. The PhD is an entry-level requirement for most faculty positions in the pharmaceutical and social and administrative sciences, and occasionally in pharmacy practice—especially if the position comes with a high research expectation.

Some positions may even require you to complete research work beyond a PhD, commonly referred to as a "post doc," to gain more experience in writing grants and publications before beginning a faculty career. Master's-level degrees are occasionally combined with a professional degree, such as a PharmD combined with an MBA or an MPH, to give the candidate unique opportunities to teach and perform scholarly activities across disciplines.

Some faculty positions at colleges of pharmacy do not require you to complete a residency, fellowship, or graduate degree to obtain a faculty appointment. Many pharmacists with first professional degrees (either the BS pharmacy or PharmD) contribute to pharmacy education by facilitating pharmacy practice laboratories or serving as preceptors for IPPEs and APPEs. These faculty members commonly hold part-time, adjunct, or even volunteer faculty appointments that provide many of the same benefits enjoyed by full-time faculty—particularly the opportunity to shape the next generation of pharmacists.

A professional degree in pharmacy is not necessary for all faculty positions at colleges of pharmacy. Given the wide scope of teaching and research that involves drug therapy, many schools are increasingly hiring faculty from disciplines outside of pharmacy, including chemists, statisticians, economists, and social and behavioral scientists.

Talk to Others

If you wish to pursue a graduate degree, talk with other people who have earned the degree you're interested in, especially faculty, so they can help you assess the challenges of obtaining the degree and describe the opportunities it creates.

Most likely, these people will tell you that getting good grades isn't the only measure of success in a graduate program. You also need an inquisitive nature to identify research questions and design projects to answer these questions. A sense of perseverance is also important to help you press on when your studies and research aren't going so well.

Conclusion

Some amount of postprofessional training or education is required for most faculty positions at a college of pharmacy. Almost everyone who has gone down this path agrees that the added costs—including time, effort, and money—are well worth the rewards.

Keep in mind that good faculty members are, by nature, willing learners. Pursuing postprofessional training or education not only opens the door to a career as a pharmacy faculty member, but enables you to continue to learn more that will benefit your teaching, scholarship, and patient care.

Where to Find More Information on Preparing for an Academic Career

Academy of Managed Care Pharmacy (AMCP) Residency Information
www.amcp.org
Click on "Professional Practice" and then "Residencies" to find accreditation standards for managed care residencies and a directory of programs.

American Association of Colleges of Pharmacy (AACP) Listing of Graduate Programs
www.aacp.org
Click on "Resources," then "Student Center," then "Graduate and Research Students" for a listing of graduate degree programs offered by schools and colleges of pharmacy in the United States.

continued on page 54

continued from page 53

American College of Clinical Pharmacy (ACCP) Residency Information
www.accp.com
Click on "Careers" to find a directory of residencies, fellowships, and graduate programs in clinical pharmacy as well as guidelines for clinical fellowship training programs.

American Pharmacists Association (APhA) Career Pathway Evaluation Program for Pharmacy Professionals
www.pharmacist.com
This program provides resources that allow pharmacists to assess their own interests and then learn about careers in pharmacy matching that interest. Many colleges of pharmacy offer the program as a live workshop for their students. Interested pharmacists can also access the materials online at the URL above and search for Career Pathway Evaluation Program.

APhA Community Pharmacy Residency Program
www.pharmacist.com
Click on "Pharmacy Practice" and then "Residencies/Advanced Training" for information about community pharmacy residencies, including accreditation standards and a directory of programs.

American Society of Health-System Pharmacists (ASHP) Residency Information
www.ashp.org
Click on "Accreditation" and then "Resident Information" for general information about pharmacy residency training programs, including accreditation standards and a directory of programs.

Chapter 5

Obtaining a Position as a Pharmacy Faculty Member

Regardless of where you are in your education, postgraduate training, or professional career, it's always good to keep your eyes and mind open to new opportunities and to consider the possibility of a career as a pharmacy faculty member.

Universities have addressed the shortage of pharmacists by creating new doctor of pharmacy programs and expanding pharmacy student enrollments at existing colleges of pharmacy. This has sparked an unprecedented demand for pharmacy faculty members. The need for pharmacy faculty is expected to remain high because of anticipated growth in the number and size of programs, as well as retirements and turnover among existing pharmacy faculty members.

The Process Takes Time

The process of obtaining a faculty position can be likened more to a marathon than a sprint. Although openings may become available at any time, many institutions start searching for candidates almost a year before the academic year in which the position will begin.

Candidates often apply in the fall and early winter, and search committees evaluate candidates and schedule interviews during the winter and spring. Often, institutions aim to make hiring decisions in the spring so they can extend an offer and negotiate details well before the faculty position begins in the fall.

Learning About Opportunities

How do you learn about faculty opportunities at colleges of pharmacy? Most likely, it won't be in the classified ads section of your local newspaper. Colleges of pharmacy actively seek highly qualified applicants through promotional activities that are likely to generate large pools of candidates who are a good match for their open positions.

Like other large employers, colleges and universities often post announcements for open faculty positions on their websites, so visiting them is a good way of learning about open positions, especially if you're focusing on a particular university or geographic

> The process of obtaining a faculty position can be likened more to a marathon than a sprint.

area. But given the degree of postgraduate training and specialization required for many faculty positions, you may find that any one particular college will not have an opening for someone with your particular training or interests at a given time. Cast a wide net and consider positions at a number of colleges of pharmacy to improve your chances of obtaining the right fit for you.

Databases and Career Resources

One way of casting a wide net is to use the employment databases provided by many professional organizations, which are searchable based on such characteristics as discipline, clinical specialty, and geographic location. Organizations that list openings for faculty positions at colleges of pharmacy include:

- American Association of Colleges of Pharmacy (AACP)
- American Association of Pharmaceutical Scientists (AAPS)
- American College of Clinical Pharmacy (ACCP)
- American Society of Health-System Pharmacists (ASHP)

Many professional organizations also offer career planning resources to members, such as:

- Guidance on résumé writing and interviewing skills.
- Placement services for open faculty positions.
- Forums at professional conferences for candidates interested in faculty positions.
- Opportunities to meet with representatives from colleges of pharmacy to learn more about their positions and to begin the application process.

Networking

Another way to learn about faculty positions is by networking with professional colleagues and coworkers. Many pharmacy faculty members first learned of their current position not from an ad in a journal or a posting on a website, but from a friend or colleague who thought that they might be interested in an opportunity. People who know you and your skills, interests, and experiences can be your best allies in your search.

College of pharmacy faculty search committees often begin their searches by developing lists of prospective candidates suggested by peers in the profession. If you are still pursuing your professional education or postgraduate training, you have great resources in your faculty, preceptors, advisors, and mentors, who are often networked with others in their fields. These networks can open doors to opportunities in ways that are usually not possible if you simply respond to a position announcement on a website.

Internal Openings

If you're a graduate student at a college of pharmacy or a pharmacist at an academic medical center, you may become aware of faculty positions that arise in your own institution. Pursuing these positions has advantages and disadvantages for internal candidates.

On the one hand, internal candidates often know the institution well and may be able to quickly learn what they'll need to do to succeed as a faculty member. On the other hand, faculty search committees often seek candidates who can bring new ideas to the faculty and may prefer candidates who were educated or trained at other institutions. Internal candidates also may have difficulty differentiating themselves from the people they trained with; that is, demonstrating how they stand out from their peers and capitalizing on their own personal reputation and uniqueness.

Learn More Before Applying

Once you identify positions of interest, you need to learn more about them as well as about the college of pharmacy and university before you contact the search committee chair or apply for the position.

Check the Website

To explore each position, start by visiting the website for each university and its college of pharmacy. Look for statements of the institution's mission and values, which give you a sense of major priorities and how the institution values teaching, scholarship, and service.

On the college of pharmacy website, pay particular attention to the department or division in which the position is based—especially the types of teaching, scholarship, and service performed by the people who will be your colleagues if you land the position.

When reviewing college and university websites, keep in mind that they highlight the school's best attributes because their primary purpose is usually marketing the institution to prospective students, faculty, alumni, donors, and community members. As a prospective faculty member, you certainly want to know what makes the school a good place to study or work, but you also want to learn about aspects of being part of the institution on a daily basis that may not be included on their website.

Talk to People

To learn more about the opportunities and challenges at a particular institution, make it a point to gather information from colleagues in your professional network. Perhaps someone you know already works for that institution or has worked there in the past. Colleagues may be acquainted with someone employed there or who is familiar with the institution.

> People who know you and your skills, interests, and experiences can be your best allies in your search.

Focus your conversations on aspects of the institution you're not likely to learn about from websites. A small sampling of questions that websites don't cover:

- What are the workload expectations for faculty, particularly regarding teaching and research?
- How well do faculty interact with each other? Is there a sense of collegiality, or competitiveness?
- What has been the turnover rate among faculty in the position and department? If the turnover rate seems high, probe further to learn more about why people have chosen to leave.
- How have promotion and tenure standards been applied to existing faculty?

Your goal at this point is to gather as much information as possible about the position and institution so you can assess the fit and develop a list of questions to ask if you choose to apply.

Reach Out to the Chair

Contact someone at the college of pharmacy—typically a department chair or search committee chair—before you submit an application so you can learn more about the position beyond its written description. Conversations with those helping to screen and select candidates give you the opportunity to raise questions and get insights so you can decide if you want to go further in the application process.

Think Long Term

Applying for a position, interviewing, and evaluating candidates is intensive and time-consuming. The hours and effort that you, the search committee, faculty interviewers, and college administrators put into the process are likely to be greater than those expended when you applied to get into college or a training program, or for that matter, applied for any other job.

Why is it so intensive? Because of the degree of commitment necessary on both sides—yours and the college's—to ensure that the position is filled with the right candidate. Unlike in most other types of jobs, faculty members are usually hired based on their potential to remain in their positions and contribute to their institution and fields throughout their professional careers. The goal of the faculty search process is creating a long-term relationship—akin to a marriage—rather than a one- or two-year partnership before you move on to something else. When you research and apply for faculty positions, ask yourself: "Can I see myself committing to this position and institution throughout my professional career?"

The Application Process

Typically, the position announcement will state what a prospective candidate needs to do to formally apply for the faculty position. Figures 5-1 and 5-2 provide sample position announcements.

Candidates are generally required to submit a cover letter and a curriculum vitae (CV). These documents are described briefly in this chapter; you can find detailed information about how to prepare them in *The Pharmacy Professional's Guide to Résumés, CVs, and Interviewing*, published by the American Pharmacists Association.

You must supply the names and contact information for several references. These references may be contacted by members of the search committee, or they may be asked to write a letter of reference on your behalf. You may also be asked to provide statements of about one to three pages summarizing your teaching philosophy and scholarly interests. These statements should be reflective, summarizing your past and present interests and philosophy and highlighting the direction you see yourself taking in the future. Many student pharmacists have had experience developing these types of reflective statements in the portfolios they developed while in pharmacy school. Put time and effort into preparing these materials so they make a good impression.

Figure 5-1 | **Sample Description for a Tenure-Track Faculty Position**

Assistant Professor of Pharmacy Administration

DEPARTMENT
Clinical and Administrative Sciences, College of Pharmacy

DUTIES AND RESPONSIBILITIES
Responsibilities are teaching, service, and research. Specifically they include:

1. Teaching required and elective courses in social and administrative pharmacy in the PharmD curriculum and pharmacy administration graduate program
2. Participating in department, college, and university committees, as well as service to the profession
3. Obtaining external funding through grants and contracts for scholarly projects
4. Publishing in peer-reviewed journals

QUALIFICATIONS
Applicants should possess a PhD in pharmacy administration or related field and have a strong background in research design and outcomes research. Familiarity with Medicaid programs and claims data highly desirable.

SALARY
Competitive and dependent on education and experience.

APPLICATIONS
Applications are invited for a 12-month tenure-track position. Send cover letter, curriculum vitae, and three references to:

Dr. Robert Pharmacist, Department Chair
Clinical and Administrative Sciences
College of Pharmacy
Telephone: (222) 765-4321
Email: chair@pharmacy.edu

Electronic submissions are encouraged. The review of applications will begin immediately and continue until the position is filled.

The College of Pharmacy is an Equal Opportunity/Affirmative Action Employer.

Figure 5-2 | **Sample Description for a Clinical-Track Position**

Assistant Clinical Professor

The School of Pharmacy at Northern Southwestern University invites applications from highly motivated candidates for a full-time Assistant Clinical Professor position with expertise in ambulatory care. This is a non-tenure-track appointment in the Department of Pharmacy Practice.

Primary responsibilities include maintenance of a clinical practice at a community health center. The faculty member will be joining an established practice site and collaborating with other faculty in the provision of clinical pharmacy services, didactic and experiential teaching, practice-based scholarship, and a PGY-1 residency program.

Qualifications
Candidates must have a PharmD degree and a residency or PharmD with equivalent clinical experience. Evidence of successful teaching is also required. Candidates must be eligible for pharmacist licensure.

Additional Information
The School of Pharmacy at Northern Southwestern strives to be the national model for education and research in the health, psychosocial, and biomedical sciences. It supports the University's mission of educating students for a life of fulfillment and accomplishment and creating and translating knowledge to meet global and societal needs.

Northern Southwestern is near several medical schools and nationally recognized medical centers. The university is located in a large metropolitan area with a variety of cultural opportunities.

Salary will be commensurate with education, training, and experience and includes an outstanding benefits package. The start date for this position is August 2010. Evaluation of candidates will begin immediately and applications will be accepted until the position is filled.

continued on page 62

Figure 5-2 | *continued from page 61*

Equal Employment Opportunity

Northern Southwestern University is an Equal Opportunity/Affirmative Action, Title IX, and ADVANCE institution. Minorities, women, and persons with disabilities are strongly encouraged to apply. Northern Southwestern University embraces the wealth of diversity represented in our community and seeks to enhance it at all levels. Northern Southwestern University is an E-Verify employer.

How to Apply

Applications must be submitted online by visiting the College website at http://www.Northern_Southwestern.edu and clicking on Faculty Positions.

Applicants should submit a formal letter of interest, along with curriculum vitae and the names and addresses of three references.

More information regarding this position may be obtained by contacting Krista Kapsule, PharmD, Professor and Chair, Department of Pharmacy Practice, at k.kapsule@Northern_Southwestern.edu.

Cover Letter

A cover letter should be a brief statement (generally no more than one page) in a standard business letter format that formally expresses your interest in being a candidate for a position. In the letter you should highlight reasons why you're a good fit for the faculty position and ways you are prepared to meet the specific job requirements described in the announcement.

Curriculum Vitae

Unlike a résumé, which is a one- or two-page document describing your education and work experience, a CV is a comprehensive listing of your education, work history, skills, and experiences pertinent to the position.

An essential document in your search for a pharmacy faculty position, your CV tells the story of your career and highlights relevant experiences. Given that pharmacy faculty members perform teaching, scholarship, and service, your CV should list activities in each category that you've carried out over the course of your education, postgraduate training, and career. At many universities, career resource centers sponsor programs to help candidates construct a good CV. Take a look at the CVs of faculty mentors for examples of format and content.

References

When you are asked to submit the names and contact information of references, the hiring institution is looking for people who have knowledge of your qualifications for the position.

References may be asked to write a letter of recommendation on your behalf, or they may be contacted by a search committee while it is evaluating the pool of candidates to learn more about your suitability for the position. Your reference will be asked to describe how you have worked together and to provide an assessment of your teaching and research, and possibly of your clinical skills and abilities.

In choosing your references, think about people you know well professionally who have a strong sense of your qualifications for the position. Ideal references would include:

> In choosing your references, think about people you know well professionally who have a strong sense of your qualifications for the position.

- Faculty with whom you have worked, such as serving as a teaching assistant in their class or taking part in a joint research project.
- Directors and preceptors of your postgraduate training programs.
- Coworkers who have worked in environments similar to that of the position for which you are applying.

Avoid the temptation to select references based on their acclaim within a field, particularly if the reference does not know you very well. If references cannot answer a wide range of questions about your qualifications, they may be more likely to hinder than help you secure a pharmacy faculty position.

The Competition

The degree of competition you can expect for a faculty position at a college of pharmacy depends on many variables, such as how many people in the market have the required background and training. As the level of expertise and specialization required for the position increases, the size of the applicant pool typically decreases.

It's not generally possible to learn the identities of other candidates for a position, but you should try to ascertain the attributes of people who would typically apply, such as level of education and training and degree of research and clinical experience.

A position description will describe the minimum level of attributes required for a position, but to truly understand the qualities and characteristics of people hired into faculty positions, get to know faculty at your institution and at institutions similar to the one you'd like to work at. You may find that some colleges are looking for new faculty with expertise in specific types of research or clinical practice. Others may seek faculty from particular types of universities or training programs.

For example, schools of pharmacy with a research-oriented mission often want faculty candidates from similarly research-oriented programs, while those with teaching-centered missions commonly seek candidates with additional teaching credentials such as a teaching-intensive residency, a teaching certificate program, or experience as a teaching assistant. Knowing these attributes can help you distinguish yourself from other applicants in your cover letter and interviews.

The Search Committee

After the college of pharmacy receives applications for a pharmacy faculty position, the applications are reviewed by a search committee consisting primarily of faculty members in the department where the position will be based. The committee assesses your cover letter and CV to determine if you seem to have the attributes necessary to succeed in the position.

At this point, members of the search committee may follow up with your references to learn more about your relevant experience and qualifications. They may also conduct a preliminary telephone interview with you to explore your communication skills, enthusiasm, professional skills, and degree of interest in the position.

The next step is for the committee to perform an initial ranking of candidates to determine which ones to invite to campus for interviews. Typically, two to five candidates are invited to interview for a pharmacy faculty position, depending on the nature of the position, size of the applicant pool, and the degree of difficulty anticipated in filling the position. If they know that the candidates in the pool are likely to apply for similar positions at other institutions, search committees may choose to interview a greater number of candidates.

The Faculty Interview

Your invitation to interview for a pharmacy faculty position gives you the opportunity to show that you're the ideal candidate. Formal interviews for faculty positions typically take place on the college campus as well as at other clinical and research sites where the candidate will work or interact.

An interview typically takes one to two days and often involves an overnight stay on or near campus. Even though it's called an "interview," it's really a series of meetings and conversations with a variety of people on and off campus. Typically, the people who will interview you over the course of your visit include:

- Faculty
- Administrators (including both the dean and department chair)
- Staff
- Students
- Clinicians
- Researchers

During these meetings, the interviewers will explore your interests, flesh out your qualifications for the position, provide information about resources offered by the college and university, and answer your questions.

If your position involves teaching and research, you will likely be asked to give a presentation during your interview. This presentation gives you the opportunity to explain your line of research and demonstrate your passion for teaching and scholarship. The presentation also gives the search committee and faculty the chance to evaluate your potential as an academician.

Keep Shining Through the Stress

Candidates for pharmacy faculty positions often find the interview process mentally and physically stressful. In addition to the pressure of answering questions—often the same questions asked multiple times by different interviewers—you may experience other sources of stress.

Travel to and from the interview site, long days of meetings with all kinds of people you've never met before, and giving what is likely one of the most important presentations of your career can all take their toll. Despite the challenges and strains, you must be resilient, continuously displaying your sincere interest in the position and focusing on how your qualifications match those needed in the position.

Ask Good Questions

The answers you give to interviewers' questions are one part of the equation; just as important are the questions you ask during your interview. Interviewers expect you to ask well-thought-out questions that show you've done your homework. A successful interview is a two-way street; it helps the college of pharmacy evaluate your suitability for the position and helps you determine whether this institution is the best fit for your personal and professional goals.

Candidates for faculty positions should develop a list of questions to ask during an interview—questions that demonstrate your interest in the position, your curiosity about the institution, and the legwork you've put into preparing for your interview. Ask some of the same questions of a variety of people to tap different perspectives and get a well-rounded picture.

> Interviewers expect you to ask well-thought-out questions that show you've done your homework.

After you complete your interview, follow up with the search committee chair and others that you met with during the interview to say thank you and gather additional information if you need it.

If you've thought of new questions since the interview, direct them to the search committee chair, who should be able to either answer them or direct you to someone who can. It may seem more efficient to send a "thank you" email to everyone you met during an interview, but a more traditional handwritten thank-you letter or card still has its place. Taking time to prepare handwritten messages adds a personal touch, displays your sincere interest, and makes a good impression with faculty and other interviewers. It is standard practice to send one letter or card to each person you met with during your visit, whether individually or in a group interview. Plan ahead by collecting business cards or writing down correct spellings, titles, and addresses during your interview.

Steps Leading to the Offer

The interview and selection process can take weeks or even months. It is exceedingly rare for a candidate to be offered a faculty position immediately after an interview. Unlike in the movies, no one is going to exclaim "You're hired!" on the spot.

Several candidates may be interviewing for this position. Depending on when your interview occurs in the search process, it may take several more weeks until each candidate has been interviewed and the committee is able to make a recommendation. Once that recommendation is made, others at the institution may need to approve the recommendation before an offer can be extended.

At the same time, search committees realize that candidates for their positions are often applying for positions at other institutions as well. Search committees want to perform a thorough review of their candidates, yet act quickly so that they don't risk losing their best candidates to offers from other institutions.

As Agreed, Check In

The wait can be stressful, but it helps if you and the search committee chair plan to share information about where each of you is in your evaluation processes. The chair should be able to give you a general idea when the interview process will be completed. It can also help to share your plans with the search committee chair, particularly if you are already being presented with competing offers. If you have a competing offer and really want to work for an institution you are still waiting to hear from, letting the search committee chair know may help expedite a decision. If you are the ideal candidate for their position, they may prepare an offer quickly so as not to lose you.

Search Committee Ranks Finalists

After all the candidates have been interviewed, the search committee will typically meet again to rank the finalists. At this time, the committee usually (but not always) recommends that a candidate from the pool of interviewees be hired for the position.

The search committee's recommendation will be forwarded to the department chair and perhaps to the dean. One of these two people will contact the selected candidate to offer the position. Being on the receiving end of this telephone call is exciting, especially if you have your heart set on the position. However, it also begins a process of negotiation and your chance to evaluate the offer.

The Negotiation Process

During the call to offer you a faculty position, the dean or chair will probably tell you the terms of the offer and, most likely, will follow up with an email that explicitly lists the terms, which generally include:

- Salary.
- Benefits.
- Descriptions of resources that will be made available, such as startup funds for researchers, travel funds, professional development support, etc.
- Job responsibilities.
- Releases from particular activities and expectations, such as a release from teaching or college service expectations for a period of time to allow the new faculty member to develop a research program or clinical practice site.

Prepare in Advance for Negotiations

The college of pharmacy's offer represents the first step in the negotiation process. Be sure to enter negotiations with a good idea of what you would like from the position based on information you received and answers to questions you asked during the application and interview process.

Start by comparing the college's offer to your expectations. Is anything out of sync with what you thought you'd be offered? If something doesn't match what you were seeking, think about how important that item is to you. It might be something you can negotiate.

Many aspects of an offer are negotiable, but other aspects are more hard and fast. For example, starting salaries for new pharmacy faculty members tend to allow little room for negotiation because most universities keep similar types of faculty within a similar salary range. New pharmacy faculty rarely receive salaries comparable to those that new pharmacy graduates receive when they go directly into pharmacy practice. However, the benefits available to faculty members such as paid time off, retirement contributions, and support for professional development are often higher than for those taking entry-level pharmacist positions.

You may have more success negotiating for resources such as research startup funds and professional development support, especially if you can justify them based on how they will benefit you, the college, and the university.

Once an offer has been tendered, be prepared to negotiate and come to an agreement within a few days. If the terms cannot be improved to your liking, the college will need to negotiate with another candidate as soon as possible. Most colleges try to conclude the negotiation process for an entry-level faculty position within 7 to 10 days.

Accept or Decline?

Once the terms of your offer have been negotiated, it's up to you to decide whether to accept. As with many job opportunities, the faculty position offering the highest salary may not necessarily be the best position for you, for a variety of reasons. You must take an introspective approach and know what is most important to you regarding:

- The position itself.
- The community in which you want to live.
- The balance you hope to achieve in your academic, professional, personal, and family life.

Declining an offer must be considered as carefully as accepting. Pharmacy academia is a very small world and candidates shouldn't apply for positions unless they truly are willing to take the position if the circumstances are right. Search committees don't like to see someone treat an interview as a "practice interview" for a position at another school of pharmacy.

However, it's possible that you may be extended an offer for a position that you realize is not a good fit for you. A college would much rather see someone turn down an offer than to have the person accept a mismatch and leave after a short time.

> Accepting an offer is the first step in building a long and professionally satisfying career as a pharmacy faculty member.

Think of it this way: accepting an offer is the first step in building a long and professionally satisfying career as a pharmacy faculty member. If the position feels wrong and you can't see yourself being happy in it, it's not for you. But if critical elements of the position line up with what you're looking for and you're excited about stepping into your new role, it's probably a good fit.

Conclusion

The process of obtaining a faculty position at a college of pharmacy is likely to be more intense than that for any other position you've considered in the pharmacy profession.

Although it can be a stressful undertaking, you need to follow the proper steps and do the appropriate research to ensure that the institution and position are a good fit for you. As with any selection process, the more information each party gathers about the other, the more likely each will arrive at an outcome with the greatest benefits in the long run.

Where to Find More Information on Obtaining a Position as a Pharmacy Faculty Member

American Association of Colleges of Pharmacy (AACP) Online Career Center

pharm.aacp.associationcareernetwork.com/Common/HomePage.aspx
Lists faculty positions offered by colleges of pharmacy across the country.

American Association of Pharmaceutical Scientists (AAPS) Career Network

www.aapspharmaceutica.com/careercenter/index.asp
Lists positions in the pharmaceutical sciences, particularly in pharmacology, toxicology, pharmaceutics, and medicinal chemistry, including faculty positions at colleges of pharmacy.

American College of Clinical Pharmacy (ACCP) Online Position Listings

www.accp.com/careers/onlinePositionListings.aspx
Lists positions in clinical pharmacy practice and research, including faculty positions at colleges of pharmacy.

American Society of Health-System Pharmacists (ASHP) Professional Placement Service (PPS)

www.careerpharm.com/employer/pps/index.aspx
Lists positions in hospital and health-systems practice, including positions with faculty appointments at colleges of pharmacy.

The Pharmacy Professional's Guide to Résumés, CVs, & Interviewing, 2nd ed.

Reinders TP. Washington, DC: American Pharmacists Association; 2006
A resource to help pharmacists and student pharmacists prepare cover letters, résumés, and curricula vitae and prepare for successful interviews.

Chapter 6

Lessons from Pharmacy Faculty

If you're getting started as a pharmacy faculty member—or even thinking about it—you can learn a lot from others who have preceded you down this path. Most people in the field are more than willing to share what they've learned and to tell you about the bits of knowledge and experience that helped them get their career off to a good start.

This chapter presents interviews with five pharmacists who have successfully navigated through pharmacy school, post-professional education or training, and an entry-level faculty position, and ultimately to successful careers as pharmacy educators.

In some ways you couldn't find five people more different from each other. Each comes from a different discipline, teaches at a different type of institution—some teaching-intensive, some research-intensive—and performs different types of functions. However, as you read their interviews, you'll also find they have much in common in how they prepared to become pharmacy faculty members, what they've done to achieve success, and the lessons they've learned along the way.

Despite their different paths, during the course of their careers they've come to recognize the importance of building relationships; discovered that sometimes journal submissions are rejected no matter how hard they worked on them, but it's all a useful learning process; and realized that teaching and mentoring bring great personal rewards.

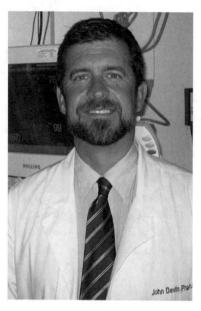

John Devlin Pharl

John W. Devlin

Associate Professor, Northeastern University, Bouvé College of Health Sciences, School of Pharmacy

In addition to his role at Northeastern, John holds an appointment as an adjunct associate professor with Tufts University School of Medicine and works as a clinical pharmacist specialist in critical care at Tufts Medical Center.

John joined the faculty at Northeastern as a tenure-track associate professor in 2003 and gained tenure in 2009. He obtained a BS in pharmacy and a PharmD from the University of Toronto. Then he completed a pharmacy practice residency at the London Health Sciences Centre in London, Ontario, and a critical care pharmacy fellowship at Henry Ford Hospital in Detroit. He is a fellow of both the American College of Clinical Pharmacy and the American College of Critical Care Medicine, and is a board-certified pharmacotherapy specialist.

Q: Talk about your educational background and training.

A: I was drawn toward a career in hospital pharmacy practice based on experiences I had while in pharmacy school. I particularly liked the environment at large teaching hospitals, which is where I gained my first exposure to clinical pharmacy practice.

During my pharmacy practice residency at the London Health Sciences Centre, I was mentored by Charlie Bayliff, PharmD, a practitioner who made it a point to have independent relationships with his patients. Dr. Bayliff was also involved in research and published many articles in the pharmacy and medical literature. During my residency I had the opportunity to contribute to a case study he published in the *Canadian Journal of Hospital Pharmacy,* which fueled my desire to develop as a writer.

I practiced pharmacy for several years in critical care and began to work with medical school faculty on their research. I realized that I needed a better understanding of the scientific foundations of clinical pharmacy practice, so I decided to complete a post-BS doctor of pharmacy degree at the University of Toronto. I followed this with a critical care pharmacy fellowship at Henry Ford Hospital in Detroit and gained both extensive research experience and the skills necessary to become an independent clinical researcher.

Q: Given your education and training, what types of positions in addition to academia did you consider?

A: After completing my fellowship, I remained in clinical practice at Detroit Receiving Hospital and University Health Center. I also held an adjunct faculty appointment at Wayne State University College of Pharmacy and Health Professions and served as director of Wayne State's Critical Care Pharmacy Fellowship Program. I focused on research and published many papers, but always felt challenged by the extensive patient care and service responsibilities that are part of any health-system-based clinical pharmacist specialist position.

Although I had academic, clinical, and research responsibilities, I felt that my position as a hospital clinical pharmacist limited my ability to fully develop a high-quality research program and enjoy the security that comes with a tenured faculty position. I knew that a tenure-track faculty position, where I could focus on developing my own research program independent of working under a physician, would be appealing. And I knew that I liked serving as a mentor to my fellows. It became clear that the time had arrived to look for positions in academia.

Q: What ultimately led you to choose a career in academia?

A: The enjoyment I got from mentoring the pharmacists in my fellowship program was a key factor. I wanted to continue working with fellows and pharmacy students and to pursue my research interests in critical care. I was drawn to Northeastern by the combination of teaching, clinical practice, and research opportunities through the school of pharmacy and the world-renowned medical centers in Boston.

I started my position by developing a clinical practice at Tufts Medical Center and a research program focused on identifying, preventing, and treating agitation and delirium in intensive care units (ICUs). My previous critical care research and publications helped me develop relationships with physicians and others at Tufts, which led to an adjunct faculty appointment with Tufts Medical School—useful in forming new research partnerships and competing for grants.

I enjoy the research but I also like teaching at Northeastern, especially my critical care advanced pharmacy practice experience and my clinical research methods course.

Q: What types of activities did you perform in the first few years of your academic career?

A: Before launching my career in academia, I'd always been on academia's periphery and had never had a formal teaching role as a lecturer. Over my first several years as a pharmacy faculty member, I learned about effective pedagogy strategies and educational assessment techniques from my colleagues at Northeastern.

> Have a strong relationship with your department chair and make sure you are both on the same wavelength regarding goal-setting and career development.

Very few members of the Pharmacy Practice Department focused on research when I started at Northeastern, but rather than let that interfere with pursuing an academic career there, I leveraged my research experience to take a leadership role within my department. I served as a resource to other department members to help them develop their own research. I also used my professional networks to help recruit additional faculty interested in performing research at academic medical centers in Boston.

Northeastern and Tufts formed a partnership to develop a critical care pharmacy fellowship program. Establishing the fellowship and serving as its director allow me to train and mentor future investigators and extend my research productivity.

Q: Which activities took more time than you expected? Which took less time?

A: Learning to balance teaching and service activities at Northeastern with patient care and research at Tufts took more time than I'd anticipated. By starting the fellowship program and bringing in a research fellow I was able to make more effective use of my time, extend my activities at Tufts, and further develop my teaching and service at Northeastern.

Q: Were any activities particularly frustrating? Particularly rewarding?

A: Before becoming a faculty member at a college of pharmacy, most of my research had been conducted at hospitals where I was employed, working with physicians and other professionals who were part of the hospital. Coming to Northeastern changed the research administration dynamic because my employer was no longer an academic medical center (Northeastern does not have its own academic medical center). Now I had to deal with matters involving subcontracts between my employer and the hospital where I carry out my research, Tufts Medical Center. The issues that arise from these relationships, such as funding, indemnity insurance, and harmonizing institutional review board (IRB) requirements, add time and complexity to the research process.

I enjoy the academic community at Northeastern. We have wide-ranging expertise in research areas similar to mine and many talented educators who mentor me. Gaining tenure has provided a sense of security, given the ever-changing environments in many hospitals and health systems.

Q: Now that you are further into your career, what, if anything, has changed about what you do now compared with when you began your career?

A: I'm more comfortable as a teacher now, and therefore I don't feel as much pressure to document the outcomes of my teaching. I'm putting more thought into deciding what research projects I want to pursue and am more at ease telling people "no" when projects aren't consistent with my goals.

Given the competing demands on my time, I was careful about how much time I spent mentoring others before I obtained tenure. Now, mentoring is part of my responsibility as a tenured, senior-level faculty member.

Q: How do you see your career evolving in the future?

A: I've never had a shortage of project ideas or funded research, but finding the personnel to help complete ICU-based investigations is a continual challenge. There are a limited number of qualified pharmacy candidates interested in focusing their careers in critical care pharmacy.

It's fair to say I'm seen as a leader among my faculty peers, but I'm not interested in pursuing a career in academic administration. I serve on a number of editorial boards for scientific journals and would like to continue to expand my efforts in this area. I'd also like more time to mentor and consult with others, using my skills and experience to help others develop their research.

Q: What words of advice do you have for a new faculty member entering your field?

- Know what is expected of you from fellow faculty members, clinicians, and researchers.

- Make sure you can deliver what is expected before making a commitment, especially with respect to your research.

- Have a strong relationship with your department chair and make sure you are both on the same wavelength regarding goal-setting and career development.

- Carve out a research niche. It's important to be recognized as an expert in a particular area. You have to develop a long-term research plan with goals to be accomplished at various points in your development.

- Strive to be seen as a vital part of your academic medical center, not simply a visitor from the college of pharmacy. Develop relationships with physicians, the pharmacy department, and others at your medical center who work in your area of expertise.

- In addition to building relationships internally, network with others (both in and outside of pharmacy) who perform research in your area of expertise in the world beyond your institution.

- Be nice, bring a sense of humor to work, and smile!

> Strive to be seen as a vital part of your academic medical center, not simply a visitor from the college of pharmacy. Develop relationships with physicians, the pharmacy department, and others at your medical center who work in your area of expertise.

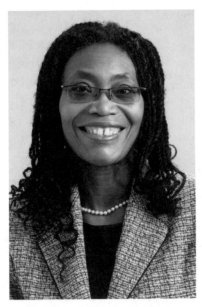

Monica Holiday-Goodman

Associate Professor of Pharmacy Administration, Department of Pharmacy Practice, College of Pharmacy, University of Toledo

Monica is also director of the Division of Pharmacy and Health Care Administration and program director of the Graduate Program in Pharmacy and Health Care Administration. She joined the faculty at Toledo as a tenure-track assistant professor in 1988 and gained tenure in 1994, along with promotion to associate professor.

Monica obtained a BS in pharmacy and a PhD in pharmacy and health care administration from Northeast Louisiana University (NLU), which is now the University of Louisiana at Monroe. While in graduate school, she was named the graduate student representative to the Louisiana Board of Regents. Monica's honors include earning the Kappa Epsilon Nellie Wakeman Fellowship and being named National Advisor of the Year by the Student National Pharmaceutical Association (SNPhA).

Q: Talk about your educational background and training.

A: While I was working on my pharmacy degree at Northeast Louisiana University, an important mentor, Buford Lively, EdD, told me I should consider going to graduate school. I did just that and remained at NLU, earning my PhD in pharmacy and health care administration in 1989.

I worked my way through graduate school by practicing as a community pharmacist. I really enjoyed the interactions with patients and picked up ideas for teaching and research projects I pursued in graduate school. If I could no longer work in academia, I feel comfortable with the idea of returning to community pharmacy practice.

Q: What ultimately led you to choose a career in academia?

A: My mother was a teacher. Ironically, I originally pursued pharmacy because I wanted a different field from my mother's. But as I progressed through pharmacy and graduate school, I realized that my personality is a good fit for the challenges and opportunities in academia.

In graduate school I worked as a teaching assistant, which gave me experience teaching in both the practice lab and the classroom. I also got involved in research and writing manuscripts with my advisor.

Q: Given your education and training, what types of positions did you consider other than academia?

> Never give up on yourself, even when things aren't going so well. Be relentless, but also realistic.

A: I briefly thought about the pharmaceutical industry, but I knew I wouldn't be comfortable in an environment where I felt I'd have to fight to justify my position every year.

Once I decided on academia, I interviewed at three colleges of pharmacy that had similar positions and expectations. Even though the University of Toledo was "up north" and the furthest from home of the three, I chose it because the people were so friendly and welcoming and it was the best fit for my personality. I started in 1989 and have been there ever since.

Q: What types of activities did you perform in the first few years of your academic career?

A: At Toledo, I got involved in teaching from the start, coordinating pharmacy administration courses and teaching pharmaceutical marketing and management. I also taught courses and advised students in Toledo's MS in pharmacy administration program. Working with graduate students enabled me to develop an active research program.

Early in my career, I received a Grant Award to Pharmacy Schools (GAPS) grant from the American Association of Colleges of Pharmacy (AACP) to fund a teaching project, as well as a grant from the Ohio Board of Regents to assess the need for pharmacy services in the Toledo metropolitan area. These grants helped jump-start my scholarly productivity. My department chair tried to protect me from taking on too much committee and service work early on. Later I revved up my service activities, but in the beginning it made sense to concentrate on teaching and scholarship, the areas most likely to earn me promotion and tenure at my institution.

Q: Which activities took more time than you expected? Which took less time?

A: Trying to obtain funding and publish manuscripts took more time than I expected. Like many new faculty, I was used to being a successful student in pharmacy and graduate school and to receiving generally positive feedback for my work. I wished I knew that getting research grant proposals and manuscripts rejected was normal, particularly for faculty members early in their careers.

Initially, these rejections upset me. I'd think, "I'm never going to publish in that journal again!" But I learned not to take it personally. This helped me improve the quality of my submissions, and over time, more of my research grant proposals and manuscripts were accepted.

I found that developing good relationships with students took less time than I anticipated. This was probably because of my teaching experience in graduate school, my experience as a pharmacist and pharmacy student (which helped me recognize what these students expect), and the words of advice my mom shared from her own years of teaching. For example, I always remember her telling me, "Don't worry about whether students appreciate you as a teacher; just do your best to give them the knowledge they need to succeed." I've learned to value that wisdom even more as I've seen my students make the transition from student pharmacist to pharmacist.

Q: Were any activities particularly frustrating? Particularly rewarding?

A: Requests for proposals (RFPs) in my field often have short turnaround times, some as little as two to three weeks, which is frustrating because I want my proposals to be high quality.

Also, now that I've received promotion and tenure, I find there's a lack of mentoring for faculty in the middle of their careers. With all the effort put into mentoring faculty before they get tenure, it's surprising that colleges sometimes forget that people who have cleared this initial hurdle still have long careers ahead of them and could use advice along the way.

Seeing students progress through the college's professional and graduate programs gives me a great deal of pride. Many of my graduate students have gone on to receive a PhD and other graduate degrees, and several now have positions in academia, government, and the pharmaceutical industry. I'm just as proud of my PharmD graduates; I love seeing them in local pharmacies doing great things for my community.

Q: What would you consider the most challenging aspect of starting your academic career?

A: I'd say it was finding a focus area for my teaching and scholarship. For the most part I was teaching the administrative and managerial aspects of pharmacy practice, but I was also interested in social and behavioral aspects of health care. Eventually I developed ways to integrate my interests. For example, I have my students create proposals for marketing pharmacy products and services to diverse populations in their communities.

The process of seeking promotion from the rank of associate professor to professor has had its trying moments. The leadership in my department has gone through several changes. Sometimes I didn't have a mentor to help advise me about what I needed to do to achieve full professor status.

As my kids get older, family takes a higher priority in my life, and that poses challenges, too.

Q: Now that you are further into your career, what, if anything, has changed about what you do now compared with when you began your career?

A: Since receiving tenure I feel I can pursue more projects I'm truly interested in rather than only those most likely to lead to my promotion. Also, I've gotten more involved in service and leadership at my college and university as well as in professional associations. This gives me the ability to advise and mentor others as they progress through their careers.

Q: How do you see your career evolving in the future?

A: I've taken on administrative responsibilities, such as serving as director of the Division of Pharmacy and Health Care Administration and director of the graduate program. I'd like to start a multidisciplinary research center focusing on health disparities and access to health care. In the near future, I hope to achieve my goal of obtaining the rank of full professor.

Q: What words of advice do you have for a new faculty member entering your field?

- Have a set of goals, along with plans for how you will achieve them. This is important not just when you start your academic career, but also when you obtain promotion and tenure and beyond.

- Keep a list or a calendar of major grant deadlines in your field. Many grants are offered on an annual cycle, but some are available more often. If you don't have time to respond to an RFP right then, keeping such a calendar will help you know when to submit for the next review cycle.

- Never give up on yourself, even when things aren't going so well. Be relentless, but also realistic.

- Always remind yourself why you wanted to pursue a career in academia. Periodically reassess your accomplishments against what you'd set out to achieve. You'll likely be pleasantly surprised by the results.

Always remind yourself why you wanted to pursue a career in academia. Periodically reassess your accomplishments against what you'd set out to achieve. You'll likely be pleasantly surprised by the results.

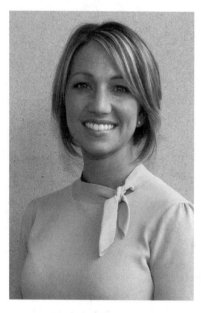

Amie Brooks

**Associate Professor, Division of
Pharmacy Practice, St. Louis College
of Pharmacy (StLCOP)**

In addition to her position as associate
professor at StLCOP, Amie practices as a
clinical pharmacist in the Family Practice
Department at the North Central Community Center and is director of StLCOP's
Ambulatory Care Residency Program.

Amie joined the faculty at Midwestern University Chicago College of Pharmacy (CCP)
as a non-tenure-track assistant professor
in 2000, at which time she established a
clinical practice at Dryer Medical Center in
Aurora, Illinois. Amie was promoted to associate professor at Midwestern in
2006 and accepted her current position at StLCOP shortly afterwards.

Amie obtained a BS in pharmacy and a PharmD from StLCOP and completed
a specialized residency in geriatric pharmacotherapy at the St. Louis Veterans
Administration Medical Center, Jefferson Barracks. She has received Best
Practice Awards from both the American Society of Health-System Pharmacists and the American Medical Group Association. Amie is a board-certified
pharmacotherapy specialist.

Q: Talk about your educational background and training.

A: As I was completing my BS in pharmacy, I felt I didn't have much knowledge
about clinical pharmacy practice. At the time I had no interest in pursuing a
career in academia.

After I received my BS in 1999, I entered StLCOP's doctor of pharmacy program, primarily because I knew that the profession was about to change to an
entry-level PharmD and I wanted to have a degree that would make me more
competitive with future graduates.

During my PharmD program, one of the faculty, Paul Dobesh, PharmD, encouraged
me to pursue a residency. I considered several programs before choosing one at
the St. Louis VA Medical Center that emphasized geriatric pharmacotherapy.

Q: What ultimately led you to choose a career in academia?

A: The first ambulatory care rotation in my doctor of pharmacy program started me on the path to an academic career. I liked the clinic activities where I could interact with patients and be directly involved in drug therapy decision-making.

At the same time I began to mentor pharmacy students on their introductory pharmacy practice experiences (IPPEs). This was the first time I felt I had something to offer in helping to educate students. My residency at the St. Louis VA Medical Center had a strong teaching development component in cooperation with StLCOP. During my residency I received formal training in teaching and was given opportunities to precept students on rotations and lead small classroom discussions.

Q: Given your education and training, what types of positions in addition to academia did you consider?

A: I considered positions other than academia, both coming out of my residency and at several other points during my career. Given my training, options included positions in ambulatory care at a hospital or clinic, or in the pharmaceutical industry as a medical science liaison. Each offered some advantages over academia, such as higher pay and a more consistent work schedule, but I always came back to the fact that academia offers benefits not found in any other practice setting.

Patient care, teaching, and scholarship are rewarding and I'm constantly challenged by the variety of my work. I also appreciate the flexibility in working arrangements that academia provides. Although I'm not on the tenure track, I feel a great sense of job security.

Q: What types of activities did you perform in the first few years of your academic career?

A: After starting my academic career at CCP I immediately took steps to lay the foundation for my career development. I had a relatively light lecture load and did not have to coordinate a course during my first year on the faculty. I also was fortunate to have been assigned lectures matching my interests and experience, especially in diabetes.

Over my first several months I developed a set of clinical pharmacy services at a medical clinic that had not previously had a clinical pharmacist. I built relationships with the medical staff before I had to precept students at my site.

I began to get involved in professional service both at CCP and in professional associations such as the American College of Clinical Pharmacy. For example, at CCP I served on the Pharmacy Practice Department Scholarship Committee, which provided resources and linked me with colleagues who would help me develop clinical practice outcomes projects at my practice site.

Q: Which activities took more time than you expected? Which took less time?

A: Taking a research project from conception to completion took much longer than I anticipated. The nature of the research I'd been involved with during my PharmD program and residency was much different than the clinical practice outcomes research I initiated as a pharmacy faculty member. Not only were my new projects more complex, often involving teams of fellow clinicians and researchers, but the outcomes I was investigating, such as changes in A1C and blood lipid levels, took longer to occur—often months or years from when the project started.

Learning how to be a good preceptor also took more time than I'd expected, as did cementing relationships with physicians and others in my clinic and building the clinical pharmacy services in which students would participate. I also discovered that it takes a great deal of time to evaluate student performance at the site and provide students with the feedback they deserve.

I've gained skills at double dipping to use time more efficiently. What I mean is, rather than viewing scholarship as something I've had to do on top of my teaching and clinical service, I have found ways to integrate scholarly activity as a natural extension of my teaching and clinical service. For example, my research evaluates the outcomes of the care I already provide to my patients. I also involve my students to help collect and evaluate the data. This extends my ability to perform clinical services and provides students with a valuable learning experience.

Q: Were any activities particularly frustrating? Particularly rewarding?

A: Establishing myself and my services at the medical clinic frustrated me at times. I had a lot of freedom because I was the one introducing clinical pharmacy services, but I had to spend time explaining and justifying them. In the end, however, being compelled to justify my services gave me the impetus to develop my clinical practice outcomes research. Starting my academic career brought so many rewards. I really liked patient care, precepting students, and giving lectures, especially answering student questions after class. Scholarship is very fulfilling too, particularly when my research projects come to fruition and are published. I've worked with a number of students on my research, many of whom have gone on to complete residencies and implement clinical pharmacy services themselves.

> Know what is expected of you, especially in terms of teaching, scholarship, and service.

Q: What would you consider the most challenging aspect of starting your academic career?

A: Trying to balance my time spent between teaching, scholarship, and service has always been a challenge. As a clinical practitioner and educator, I've had to reconcile the fact that I have at least two "bosses"—one at the clinic, the other at the college—and both have expectations for my time and activities. I've found it's important to understand exactly what's expected of me in both places and to make sure that each "boss" understands the demands placed by the other.

I struggled to find a balance between my work and my personal life. I'm fortunate to have friends and colleagues who share my professional goals and understand my struggles. I've prioritized my professional goals to help me determine when I should say yes to an opportunity.

Q: Now that you are further into your career, what, if anything, has changed about what you do now compared with when you began your career?

A: I'm making efforts to live a bit more, work a bit less, and spend more time with family—choices I can make now because of the work I did earlier in my career. By creating niches for myself in both scholarship and teaching, I now have the chance to do interesting things and I feel a greater sense of control. For example, I'm now the director of StLCOP's Ambulatory Care Residency Program, which I enjoy.

Q: How do you see your career evolving in the future?

A: I'd like to conduct more clinical outcomes research projects, particularly in diabetes management, lead more committees at my college and in professional organizations, and be a mentor to faculty. I don't necessarily see myself becoming an academic administrator, but it's rewarding to share what I've learned with faculty early in their professional development.

Q: What words of advice do you have for a new faculty member entering your field?

- Know what is expected of you, especially in terms of teaching, scholarship, and service, and develop a good relationship with your department chair, vice chairs, and other leaders in your department.

- Don't wait to get started on your scholarship activities. If you feel you need more research skills, seek development opportunities. Learn to double dip by getting scholarship out of your teaching and clinical service.

- Seek mentors from both within and outside of your discipline.

- Get involved, both at the college and professional levels. The networks you form early in your career will pay great dividends later.

- When you face challenges, remember why you wanted to go into academia in the first place!

> Get involved, both at the college and professional levels. The networks you form early in your career will pay great dividends later.

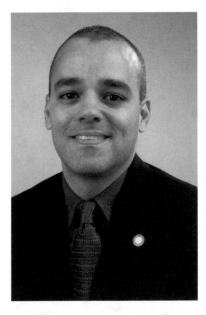

José Manautou

Associate Professor of Toxicology, Department of Pharmaceutical Sciences, School of Pharmacy, University of Connecticut

José obtained a BS in pharmacy from the School of Pharmacy at the Medical Sciences Campus of the University of Puerto Rico. He went on to complete a PhD in pharmacology and toxicology from the School of Pharmacy and Pharmaceutical Sciences at Purdue University.

José joined the University of Connecticut as a tenure-track assistant professor in 1995 and gained tenure and promotion to associate professor in 2001. A leading authority on acetaminophen hepatotoxicity, José's research has resulted in hundreds of peer-reviewed papers and presentations. He has been invited to serve on many editorial boards and review panels for the National Institutes of Health (NIH). José is a fellow of the Academy of Toxicological Sciences and is currently the Marlene L. Cohen and Jerome H. Fleisch Scholar at the University of Connecticut.

Q: Talk about your educational background and training.

A: I was always intrigued by biology and how the body works, but wasn't really interested in going to medical school, so I decided on pharmacy school at the University of Puerto Rico. My courses interested me tremendously. While earning my BS degree I took advantage of opportunities to work as an undergraduate teaching assistant and to do research. I was selected to participate in a summer research internship program at Purdue University's School of Pharmacy and Pharmaceutical Sciences, where I performed research in pharmacology and toxicology. As I continued my BS studies I began working in community and hospital pharmacies as a student intern, but I knew I wanted to get back into the lab. This led me back to Purdue to pursue a PhD with an emphasis in toxicology.

After completing my PhD in 1991 I considered postdoctoral research positions in the pharmaceutical and consumer products industries, which is where many toxicology PhD graduates pursue their careers. However, a researcher from the University of Connecticut School of Pharmacy, Steven Cohen, PhD, came to Purdue to give a seminar on acetaminophen toxicity, an area of research that intrigued me. I felt that the environment at the University of Connecticut would provide me with ample opportunities to develop my research.

Q: What ultimately led you to choose a career in academia?

A: During my postdoctoral work I helped train others in my lab and I was given the chance to lecture in graduate-level toxicology courses. I felt very comfortable in a college of pharmacy environment. My mentors saw my leadership traits and my potential as a faculty member, and they encouraged me to pursue a career in academia.

Q: Given your education and training, what types of positions in addition to academia did you consider?

A: My initial inclination had been to go into industry, the most common path for those with my background, but after interviewing for several positions, I felt that industry was too "corporate." I wanted the freedom to expand my scientific base and pursue new lines of research.

When I decided on academia, I considered several positions before deciding to stay at the University of Connecticut's pharmacy school as an assistant professor. I was somewhat concerned about remaining at the same school where I did my postdoctoral work, since it's important to be able to establish a reputation independent of the researchers I worked with during my post doc. In the end, I felt that staying at the University of Connecticut was the best fit for me.

Q: What types of activities did you perform in the first few years of your academic career?

A: During my first year on the faculty I didn't do much teaching. As a tenure-track faculty member at a research-intensive university, I knew that it would be important to set up a lab, perform experiments, and publish my research. Eventually I took on more responsibilities in teaching and service. By my second year on the faculty I was asked to teach a large portion of a pharmacology course. Rather than depend on the former professor's old notes, I wrote an entire semester's worth of lectures from scratch.

> Create a line of expertise, or niche, for yourself— a particular type of work that people can associate you with.

I was named the coordinator of a departmental seminar series, and largely because of my background as a pharmacist, was asked to be the advisor to the pharmacy school's Academy of Student Pharmacists (ASP) chapter of the American Pharmacists Association (APhA), a position I still hold.

Q: Which activities took more time than you expected? Which took less time?

A: Because I did my postdoctoral work where I began my academic career, I felt it was important to differentiate myself and my research from that of others in my department. I devoted much time to carving out a niche in a new area of research expertise.

On the other hand, preparing lectures and teaching took less time than I'd anticipated, I think because of my background as a pharmacist and my training at colleges of pharmacy. I understood right from the start how pharmacy students think and how they like to have this particular type of material delivered.

Q: Were any activities particularly frustrating? Particularly rewarding?

A: Getting my own lab ready was a bit frustrating, primarily because I'd always worked in laboratories that were already established. But even more frustrating was writing grants and research manuscripts. Many of mine were rejected early in my career, but I grew more comfortable with my work being scrutinized and I learned a lot from the reviewers' feedback, which helped me write better grants and papers. Eventually more of them were funded and published.

The academic freedom to be a scholar is wonderful. In academia you can generally pursue any type of research you are interested in as long as you can gain the funding and resources necessary to support your work. I enjoy teaching, too—being in a classroom, getting through to students, and helping students understand the material.

Q: What would you consider the most challenging aspect of starting your academic career?

A: It would have to be establishing an independent identity as a researcher. To do this, I needed to avoid distractions that could keep me from my research. At the same time, I knew it was important for my colleagues to see me as a team player, especially with respect to teaching and service. I figured out how to strategically say "yes" to some opportunities and "no" to others, especially those that could distract me from my research goals.

Q: Now that you are further into your career, what, if anything, has changed about what you do now compared with when you began your career?

A: I'm still very productive in my research but spend very little time performing it at the lab bench. Instead I plan experiments and teach my students and postdoctoral researchers how to perform the work.

> Make sure that a good faculty mentoring program is in place, either from your department chair or from senior faculty.

I also spend much more time involved in service, particularly in scientific and professional associations. I serve on editorial boards for journals in my field and on grant review panels, which gives me the opportunity to provide direction to future research in my field. I travel all over the world to present the results of my research. The professional opportunities I'm getting at this point in my career are largely due to the research I published earlier.

Q: How do you see your career evolving in the future?

A: I'll stay involved in research, but my role will probably change to focus more on mentoring others. I may not perform my own research as much. I see myself as a scientist-educator, and I still enjoy teaching in the classroom and the lab.

In directing a productive research laboratory, I've developed administrative skills that could benefit me in many ways, particularly in pursuing leadership roles at a college of pharmacy. I haven't decided if I want to take that route but am happy to know it's an option.

Q: What words of advice do you have for a new faculty member entering your field?

- It's very important to create an identity that is independent of your mentors, particularly if you stay at an institution where you trained.

- It's also essential to create a line of expertise, or niche, for yourself— a particular type of work that people can associate you with.

- Make sure that a good faculty mentoring program is in place, either from your department chair or from senior faculty.

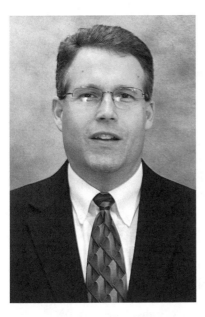

James McAuley

Associate Professor and Director of Teaching and Learning, Division of Pharmacy Practice and Administration, The Ohio State University (OSU) College of Pharmacy

Jim also holds an appointment as an associate professor in the Department of Neurology at The Ohio State University College of Medicine. Jim joined the faculty at OSU as a tenure-track assistant professor in 1993 and gained tenure and promotion to associate professor in 2001. He earned a BS and PhD in pharmacy from the University of Pittsburgh.

Jim's primary research area is epilepsy. His research has resulted in numerous peer-reviewed papers and presentations, as well as extensive service with the American Epilepsy Society and the Epilepsy Foundation of America. He is a fellow of the American Pharmacists Association and was recently named Preceptor of the Year at the OSU College of Pharmacy.

Q: Talk about your educational background and training.

A: I liked chemistry and worked in a pharmacy during high school, then enrolled in the pharmacy school at the University of Pittsburgh, graduating with a BS degree in 1987. While in pharmacy school I needed a part-time job, so I did data entry for Patricia Kroboth, PhD, who later became my mentor and graduate advisor. These experiences led me to stay at the University of Pittsburgh and enter its clinical pharmaceutical scientist PhD program, where the emphasis was on translating basic science from the bench to the bedside and back.

Q: What ultimately led you to choose a career in academia?

A: I gained a great deal from working as a teaching assistant in graduate school. Most people with a PhD in my field pursue careers in the pharmaceutical industry, but I decided to concentrate my job search on academia. As I completed my PhD, I obtained a Springboard to Teaching Fellowship from the American Foundation for Pharmaceutical Education (AFPE), which provided research funding upon my taking a position at a college of pharmacy. I became an assistant professor at The Ohio State University College of Pharmacy.

Q: What types of activities did you perform in the first few years of your academic career?

A: I immediately became immersed in teaching. Although I'd been a teaching assistant in graduate school, I now had to develop therapeutics course lectures for delivery to large groups of students. I was also responsible for leading small-group discussions, precepting pharmacy students, and conducting a research seminar.

> Find a good mentor, or even better, several mentors, such as one for teaching, another for research, and so on.

I pursued lines of research in neurology and epilepsy that I'd first identified while completing my dissertation. At OSU I started out doing lab research, but eventually transitioned my research to clinical settings, which allowed me to combine my teaching and scholarly interests. I also started getting involved in service at the college and university levels, becoming a reviewer for the university's Institutional Review Board and joining the Honors and Undergraduate Research Committee.

Q: Which activities took more time than you expected? Which took less time?

A: Getting established as a researcher took a great deal of time and effort. Unlike in graduate school, where you typically work with a team of researchers who have similar interests, I had to start new projects, identify collaborators, and write grant proposals at a new university where I didn't know many other researchers and they didn't know about my interests.

My transition to college and professional service was reasonably smooth. I connected with graduate students by volunteering to serve as a dissertation committee member and got to know colleagues by serving on various college committees. I'm also co-advisor of OSU's APhA-Academy of Student Pharmacists chapter.

Q: Were any activities particularly frustrating? Particularly rewarding?

A: I encountered certain bumps in the road to getting my research established. I put in countless hours, especially on evenings and weekends, writing manuscripts and research grant proposals, only to have many get rejected. I learned about perseverance and started to make good progress.

I get my greatest rewards from working with students. I interact with them in the classroom, at my practice site, in my research, and in extracurricular activities such as APhA-ASP. It feels great to play a role in the transition from student pharmacist to pharmacy practitioner.

Q: What would you consider the most challenging aspect of starting your academic career?

A: I had to deal with the pressure of the tenure clock and had about five or six years to prove myself as a teacher, a service provider, and a scholar at a university with a significant research mission. I worked with my department chair and had a sense of how I was progressing, but the promotion and tenure process was somewhat nebulous because many people other than my direct supervisor were involved. I found outlets for my stress by exercising and spending time with my family.

Q: Now that you are further into your career, what, if anything, has changed about what you do now compared with when you began your career?

A: In many ways, my career hasn't changed much since before I received promotion and tenure. I'm still very involved in teaching, scholarship, and service. Now that I've successfully attracted grant funding and gotten my research published, even more research opportunities have emerged, which in turn lead to more funding and publications. And more doors have opened for collaborating with others.

Now I spend time sharing my teaching and research expertise with others, particularly by mentoring new faculty. I've participated in a leadership development program at OSU that is aimed at shaping the talents of mid-career faculty. These experiences, combined with my teaching interests, led to joining my department's administrative team as the director of teaching and learning.

Q: How do you see your career evolving in the future?

A: Given my role on the department's administrative team, I may explore other administrative opportunities, such as becoming a department chair or an assistant or associate dean. However, I want to continue performing the activities that have always brought me the greatest personal satisfaction—teaching in the classroom and seeing patients in the epilepsy clinic.

Q: What words of advice do you have for a new faculty member entering your field?

- Find a good mentor, or even better, several mentors, such as one for teaching, another for research, and so on.

- Make good use of the professional development resources provided by your university.

- Have a plan and use it to say "yes" to some opportunities and "no" to others.

- Jump at opportunities to peer-review manuscripts for journals and grant proposals in your field. This will help make you a better writer for your own manuscripts and grant proposals.

- View teaching not only as a means of transmitting knowledge to students, but also as an opportunity for scholarship. Apply the scientific method to your teaching—experiment, assess and evaluate, reach and publish conclusions—just as you do in your lab or clinic.

> Jump at opportunities to peer-review manuscripts for journals and grant proposals in your field. This will help make you a better writer for your own manuscripts and grant proposals.

Chapter 7

Keys to Starting an Academic Career

Getting started as a pharmacy faculty member can be one of the most exciting times of your professional career. Whether you're relatively new to pharmacy or an experienced professional, becoming a faculty member will open many opportunities in all aspects of your life.

At the same time, starting down any new career path can be stressful and challenging. The road ahead may be fraught with pitfalls, some minor, some with the potential to hinder the development and enjoyment of your career and to interfere with your work–life balance.

The faculty members interviewed in Chapter 6 provided excellent advice for anyone considering a career in academic pharmacy. In this chapter I give my personal perspective as someone with more than 25 years of experience as both a pharmacist and educator. I hope these insights add to your success as you launch and maintain your career.

Lessons from My Path

My first glimpse at a career as a pharmacy educator began while I was a student pharmacist at the University of Wisconsin School of Pharmacy. Like most of my classmates, I assumed that I'd go into community or hospital pharmacy practice, or perhaps to another professional program such as medical school.

Becoming a pharmacy educator did not enter my mind until my second professional year when I took a course that required me to either write a paper or perform a research project. Most of my classmates chose to write the paper, but another student and I decided to conduct the research project. Up to that point, much of my experience with research involved a laboratory, and based on those experiences, I'd concluded that a career performing research really wasn't for me. However, this class project involved developing a questionnaire to gather data from pharmacists to evaluate hypotheses about whether activity in professional organizations in pharmacy school resulted in professional organization activity as pharmacists.

Working with one of my professors, Jeanine Mount, PhD, I learned that the principles of scientific research are just as important to performing good social science investigations as they are to laboratory research. Carrying out this research also engaged my intellectual curiosity. Asking well-developed questions allowed us to help explain phenomena and then apply the results of our research to create new questions for future research.

Open Mind Leads to Growth

Our choice to do a research project instead of writing a paper brought us fantastic benefits, such as the opportunity to present our results at two national pharmacy conferences and coauthor a paper for publication—fairly unusual activities for pharmacy students. It was exciting, and I wanted to learn more about research and what we can glean from research outcomes.

The most important lesson I learned at this point was to start every new experience, such as pharmacy school or a new job, with an open mind about where it might take you. Recognizing that pharmacists in academia can be researchers as well as teachers and practitioners prompted me to start considering a career as a pharmacy faculty member.

> Start every new experience, such as pharmacy school or your career path, with an open mind about where it might take you.

Leadership Roles a Plus

Several other events in pharmacy school steered me toward an academic career. I was fortunate to be elected president of our American Pharmacists Association (APhA)-Academy of Student Pharmacists (ASP) chapter, and later to be elected the ASP Region IV delegate.

Through these leadership roles, I met and learned from many other student leaders, faculty, professional association leaders, and staff. I even had opportunities to work with university administrators and elected officials, including University of Wisconsin Chancellor Donna Shalala and Wisconsin Governor Tommy Thompson, both of whom would go on to become secretary of the United States Department of Health and Human Services. Many of my fellow ASP national officers and regional delegates were considering careers in academia, which allowed us to learn from each other's interests and experiences.

Guided by Mentors

Many people mentored me in pharmacy school, but one stands out in terms of guiding me toward an academic career: Joseph Wiederholt, PhD, our ASP chapter advisor and professor of pharmacy administration. I was inspired by the energy Joe brought to his teaching, research, and interactions with students. He was very approachable, not just on matters related to ASP, but also regarding pharmacy management, which was quickly becoming my favorite subject. I would come to him with my observations and ideas based on what he was teaching, and he would always engage me in discussion about how the course topics impacted the profession, and how these topics could be better evaluated and explored through research.

When faculty members have these types of discussions with students, they commonly refer to them as "light bulb" moments: when the student begins to truly understand the concepts being taught in the classroom, lab, or practice site. Many feel that these moments are one of the most rewarding aspects of being a pharmacy faculty member.

Joe taught me that being a pharmacy educator is professionally challenging and rewarding—and also can be a heck of a lot of fun. Our hard work in the classroom and in our research often led to a lot of laughs and socialization outside the workplace. I learned an important lesson from this experience. Share your energy and passion for your chosen field with your students. Let it guide your interactions with them and the others with whom you work. You never know who may be inspired to follow your path.

During my final year of pharmacy school I had the opportunity to continue performing research with Dr. Mount, take elective courses, and tutor classmates in pharmacy management. Three years after starting pharmacy school, I had a pretty good idea that a career as a faculty member at a college of pharmacy would be a good fit for me. I knew I'd have to continue on to graduate school, where I would not only learn more about pharmacy administration and management, but also about the skills I would need to function independently as a researcher.

Some faculty members advise students interested in residencies, fellowships, or graduate school to pursue post-professional training immediately after completing their BS or first professional degree. In many cases this is good advice, because you're still in "student and learner mode," and it can be difficult to return to student life once you enter pharmacy practice and get used to the lifestyle that comes with a pharmacist's salary.

Pharmacy Practice Sparked Research Ideas

In my case, I obtained my pharmacist license and worked in a chain community pharmacy practice for two years before entering graduate school. One reason was financial. I was grateful that I'd been able to attend pharmacy school without taking on student loans or credit card debt, and I wanted to save money so I could do the same in graduate school. The decision to save money and minimize personal debt paid great dividends as I progressed through my life and career. Not only did it allow me to purchase a home shortly after finishing graduate school, but it also gave me the ability to make career decisions later based on what was best for my professional development, not simply what position paid the most.

Another reason was that I felt I still had a lot to learn about pharmacy and becoming a pharmacist. I discovered that the pharmacists, technicians, and patients at the pharmacy where I practiced after graduation were great to learn from, teaching me things that simply could not be learned in the classroom or laboratory. For example, counseling the mother of a sick child in a pharmacy is quite different from the simulation experiences I had in pharmacy practice lab when I was a student pharmacist.

My on-the-job education was particularly important given my interest in pharmacy management. Practically every idea I had for research projects in graduate school and the early part of my academic career arose from management-related questions I'd encountered in pharmacy practice. For instance, I'd noticed that patients were much more likely to accept a pharmacist's recommendation for a generic medication for some categories of drugs than for others, and I was able to turn this observation into a research project in graduate school.

Many of the concepts I currently teach in the classroom are backed up with examples of how I applied those concepts while managing a pharmacy myself. I learned that the experiences you have both inside and outside the classroom and laboratory are vitally important to your development as a pharmacy faculty member.

Reputation and Cost Key Factors in Program Choice

When the time came to return to graduate school, I considered many factors in choosing which program to attend. The reputation of the program and success of its graduates was important. Because I was planning on a career as a college of pharmacy faculty member, I wanted to learn about opportunities to develop as a teacher and researcher in graduate school. I also wanted to learn about the career paths taken by graduate students after they left the program.

Another factor influencing my program selection was the total cost of obtaining a degree, which varies depending on the graduate program. Tuition itself may be higher in graduate school than in undergraduate or professional programs, but opportunities exist to greatly reduce the cost, such as working as a teaching or research assistant or taking advantage of scholarships, fellowships, or tuition waivers. Although the University of Wisconsin has an outstanding graduate program in social and administrative pharmacy, I chose to enroll in the Division of Pharmaceutical Administration at The Ohio State University College of Pharmacy. Ohio State offered me a generous tuition waiver and teaching assistant stipend, but the primary reasons I chose their program are spelled out in the next section.

Learning from New People, New Experiences

Regardless of whether you are pursuing a residency, fellowship, or graduate degree, a common bit of advice is to seek out a different institution for your postprofessional training from the one where you received your BS or PharmD degree. Pursuing your postgraduate experience at a different institution will expose you to new ways of thinking, learning, and solving problems. Later on, you'll be well equipped to apply the best of what you learned in your undergraduate, professional, and postprofessional education to new situations you'll encounter as a faculty member.

"Light bulb" moments, when students begin to truly understand concepts, are one of the most rewarding aspects of being a pharmacy faculty member.

Obtaining your postgraduate training at a different institution also expands your professional network, adding new friends and colleagues who will play an important role throughout the rest of your career.

Postprofessional training programs can be a great way to explore different parts of the country and learn from people from other cultures and backgrounds. You're likely to find that much of your learning will occur outside of the classroom, laboratory, and practice site.

The Ohio State University had a solid program in pharmaceutical administration and a reputation for a high percentage of its graduates pursuing careers in academia. I found that my doctoral advisor (Dev Pathak, DBA) and other faculty served not only as my teachers, but also as advisors and mentors as I progressed through the program.

Learning from my fellow graduate students was another plus. Some of these students had backgrounds that were similar, but others were very different—coming from fields other than pharmacy or having pharmacy backgrounds from other countries. Each graduate student contributed to my education, and the camaraderie we developed was unlike anything I had experienced while pursuing my pharmacy degree. My fellow graduate students have remained an important part of my personal and professional network, and I'm proud to say that many have gone on to significant records of accomplishment as pharmacy faculty members themselves.

Know What You Want from Life and Career
Postprofessional programs often start with a large amount of coursework, simulations, and other supervised experiences designed to develop your knowledge and expertise. Gradually you have more time for research or patient care, and by the end of the program you demonstrate the ability to function independently as a researcher or clinician.

You will likely need a greater sense of perseverance and continuous self-motivation to complete graduate school and postprofessional programs as compared with completing undergraduate school, where you're awarded a degree after completing a defined curriculum of courses. At times, when the going got tough in graduate school, I was tempted to quit and return to pharmacy practice. However, I knew I wouldn't be able to obtain a pharmacy administration faculty position at a college of pharmacy without a PhD degree, and my desire to achieve my career goal motivated me to persevere through the ups and downs of graduate school. I briefly contemplated using my research skills in a position with the pharmaceutical industry or a managed care organization, but I learned while I was a student pharmacist and graduate student that I'm not satisfied doing just one thing. I wanted the combination of teaching, scholarship, and service that a faculty position offers.

As I was completing my dissertation research on factors that explain and predict the financial performance of community pharmacies, I began applying for a faculty position at colleges of pharmacy. Without going into the details of my search, I can tell you that getting started was probably the most difficult part of the process because it required me to be introspective and assess what was important to me. How did I want to spend my working hours and my personal time? Did I want a position that placed more emphasis on research or on teaching? How did I feel about taking a position at a new college of pharmacy as opposed to an existing program? What parts of the country would I be willing to live in? Where would I *not* want to live? What opportunities were there for my spouse? I talked at length with my mentors to evaluate each open

Lessons from My Path to Launching an Academic Career

- Keep an open mind and try new things.
- Take on leadership roles in school.
- Seek input and feedback from mentors.
- Decide whether going directly to graduate school is right for you.
- Choose a graduate program that's aligned with your goals and priorities.
- Expand your professional network.
- Learn from fellow graduate students.
- Clarify what you want from life and career.

faculty position in pharmacy administration and determine just how well the position would fit my needs and desires.

I ended up applying for five positions, getting three interviews, receiving two job offers, and accepting a position at Midwestern University Chicago College of Pharmacy (CCP), which at the time was a brand-new program that had just admitted its first class of students.

I learned from this process just how important it is to know what you want in your career and in your personal life. I used what I had discovered about myself over the years to help guide me through the application process, interviews, and evaluation of competing job offers.

I arrived at CCP in 1993 as an entry-level assistant professor of pharmacy administration and stayed 14 years until I left to take a department chair position at another institution in 2007. I was promoted twice at CCP, from assistant to associate professor and then to full professor, and I received tenure. I also helped to develop many curricular and postprofessional programs and gained experience as an administrator, both as a vice chair of my department and as a coordinator of three community pharmacy residency programs. Looking back, I can see that starting my career at CCP was a good choice for me.

To Succeed, You Must Manage Many Things

I learned many things during my start as a pharmacy faculty member that helped in my development. Following are some tips that should help you, regardless of the type of academic institution you decide to work in or your area of expertise.

Manage Expectations

What will be expected of you? This is something you should explore during the interview process and reaffirm immediately upon your arrival as a new pharmacy faculty member.

Chances are, you'll start your position with a great deal of enthusiasm. However, if you don't know how best to channel the energy you bring to the position, you are less likely to achieve the success you and your institution are hoping for.

As described in Chapter 2, colleges of pharmacy vary in the balance of teaching, scholarship, and service they expect from new faculty members. Some will release faculty from teaching and service expectations early in their careers so they can focus on scholarship; others will do just the opposite, expecting large amounts of teaching and service with relatively little time for scholarship. Knowing the balance and timing of these expectations is critical to achieving success at your institution.

It's also important to understand your institution's performance expectations in each area. This can be difficult given the variations inherent in most faculty work. Although your college's or university's faculty handbook may use terms like "excellence," "exceptional," and "acceptable" to describe levels of performance necessary to achieve promotion and tenure, you must recognize just what these terms mean in the context of what you will be expected to do.

You'll likely find that many department chairs and administrators are uncomfortable using numbers to set performance standards, such as "two peer-reviewed publications per year is 'acceptable,'" because so many factors influence these results. A simple numeric measure is almost meaningless. At the same time, however, administrators should be able to give you guidance on a regular basis. You should expect feedback at least yearly, and more often if necessary, on the extent to which your performance is meeting expectations set by your department colleagues, institution, and peers in the field.

Make it a point to understand the process by which you will be evaluated for promotion and tenure very early in your career. Learn the roles of administrators and colleagues at your institution and of peers at other institutions in determining whether you will ultimately meet promotion and tenure expectations.

You also need to recognize the connections between feedback you receive on a regular basis from students, colleagues, and administrators via teaching evaluations, annual performance reviews, and the promotion and tenure process at your institution. Few things are more frustrating for new faculty members than experiencing a disconnect between the regular feedback they receive, particularly from a direct supervisor, and how they will eventually be evaluated for promotion and tenure.

Manage Relationships

Managing your work relationships is an essential key to success. As you begin your position, the most important relationship to manage will be with your direct supervisor, which at most colleges of pharmacy will be your department chair.

Department Chair

You probably developed a relationship with your department chair during the recruitment and interview process. As your direct supervisor, your department chair can help you understand the nuances, complexities, and politics of your college or university. Most department chairs orient newly hired faculty to their departments and to the college, a process that can include formal reviews of policies and procedures as well as informal tours of buildings and introductions to colleagues.

Think of your department chair as the first source of information if you have questions. If your department chair doesn't know the answer, he or she will almost certainly be able to refer you to someone who does.

Department chairs often have formal roles that are important to your development as a new faculty member. They often set the workload expectations for faculty in their departments, especially the number of courses or lectures you will teach, the number of students you are expected to precept on introductory and advanced pharmacy practice experiences, and the number of professional or graduate students you will be expected to advise. Actual assignments of workload may vary; some department chairs will assign courses, lectures, and students to their faculty, while others allow new faculty to find their own assignments as long as they are within general workload expectations.

One function your department chair is almost certain to carry out is assessing your performance as a faculty member. Your chair will probably conduct a formal evaluation of your performance annually, but you should make efforts to meet with him or her more often to discuss performance expectations and assessment. The feedback your chair provides should be consistent with the expectations of other faculty members who perform similar types of work and in line with the tenure guidelines set by the college and university.

In addition to conducting the annual performance evaluation, most department chairs will be asked to assess your performance as you enter the promotion and tenure process. Others likely to play a role in evaluating your candidacy for promotion and tenure are your peers within your college, your college dean, and your provost or other administrators in your university.

Other Administrators

If your department is particularly large or includes a variety of specialists, there may be one or more vice chairs or assistant chairs in addition to the department chair. Make sure that you understand the functions these people perform and the reporting relationships between the chair, vice chairs, and department faculty.

For example, some faculty may have a first-line reporting relationship to a vice chair, who then reports to the department chair. Other vice chairs simply support the department and its chair by performing roles such as faculty development, assessment, or operations management; they may not have a formal reporting relationship with faculty.

Colleges and universities have many key administrators, including the university president and provost, as well as administrators within your college of pharmacy, such as the dean, assistant and associate deans, program directors, director of experiential education, etc. Even if you report directly to a department chair, you will have relationships with other academic administrators, especially those at the college level.

For example, if you precept student pharmacists, you may receive your assignments from a director of experiential education, who may also be involved in assessing your precepting performance. If both your department chair and other administrators are assigning you tasks and evaluating your performance, make sure that you understand how they work together to provide you with a single set of expectations.

Faculty Colleagues

Given the collegial nature of teaching, scholarship, and other faculty work, it is important to develop relationships with your faculty colleagues as you begin your new position. Faculty colleagues likely played an important role in evaluating your candidacy and deciding that the position should be offered to you. They expect that you have the skills and experience to succeed and to make positive contributions to the mission and goals of your department, college, and university.

Most of your new colleagues will be more than happy to help you, especially as you take on teaching, scholarship, and service responsibilities you may not have had in the past. You can learn a great deal from your colleagues, whether they are experienced educators and researchers or new faculty also beginning their careers.

However, you may have to take the initiative to ask your colleagues for assistance and advice. They probably won't want to presume that you need help, and they will be busy with their own responsibilities. Once you build a bridge by asking for help, don't be surprised if your colleagues request your help and advice in return.

> Take the initiative to ask colleagues for assistance and advice. Building a positive reputation becomes increasingly important as you move forward in your career.

Keep in mind that your faculty peers will probably be involved in assessing your performance at various points in your career. This may be a relatively informal process, such as a formative peer review of your teaching—that is, giving you direct feedback to help you improve—or a more formal approach in which colleagues give your department chair feedback to use in your annual review. Your faculty colleagues are also likely to play a role in your future promotion and tenure by being part of your college or university's promotion and tenure committee.

Administrative Staff

Building relationships with administrative staff may be something new for faculty members who are just getting started. The staff includes administrative assistants, personnel in student service, finance and budget, human resources, building maintenance, and other services, and every other person whose job doesn't directly involve teaching but who supports day-to-day operations.

Learning to work with administrative staff can be a new challenge for many faculty members, if for no other reason than that the services these people provide were not directly available to you when you were still pursuing your undergraduate and graduate studies. Take time to discover more about who these individuals are, what they do, and what they don't do. Once you have a grasp of their roles, they can help you perform your job more efficiently.

Ideally, your department, college, and university have enough administrative staff with the right skills so that faculty members can spend their time on the functions they are best trained for—especially teaching, scholarship, faculty governance, and service to the profession. How functions are defined between "faculty" and "staff" can vary greatly depending on your institution—yet another good reason to learn more about these roles when you start your position.

Students

Often, the most rewarding and demanding relationships new faculty members have are with their students. On one hand, the opportunity to work with students in the classroom, laboratory, or practice site is the reason why most professionals choose to pursue careers in academia. A tremendous amount of a faculty member's efforts go into preparing to interact with students, and the results of these efforts are almost universally positive.

Unfortunately, sometimes interactions between students and faculty are less than positive. You have to recognize such situations and take steps to deal with them effectively on a case-by-case basis. Examples of possible problems include incidents of uncivil behavior—ranging from passive incivilities in which students come late to class or fail to pay attention, to more overt incivilities such as vulgar language, direct threats, or sexual harassment.

Know your college's policies and procedures for handling these incidents and learn from the experiences of your peers. A highly recommended resource for pharmacy educators is *Promoting Civility in Pharmacy Education*, edited by Bruce Berger, PhD.

Academic assessment is another common source of conflict between new faculty members and students. Evaluation is an essential component of teaching and learning and is especially important in health professional programs because patients may face adverse consequences if a student's performance is sub-par. At some point, every educator has had to deal with a student whose understanding of the material did not meet the educator's expectations. The best way to minimize conflict in these situations is to clearly state the level of performance you expect from students, and present your expectations in a variety of formats, ranging from the course syllabus to the instructions on an assignment or exam.

Subjective assessments, such as grading a written paper or evaluating performance on a clinical exam, are especially susceptible to students' misperceptions of expectations. It's helpful to develop and share rubrics with students that provide examples of levels of performance associated with particular scores or grades.

Setting appropriate boundaries with students can also be an issue for new pharmacy faculty members, especially when there is a small age difference. Student pharmacists often think of young faculty members more as peers than as experienced educators, researchers, and health care professionals. You need to establish yourself as an experienced professional in the eyes of your students. Act and dress professionally and be cautious about the way you interact with students outside of the classroom. A litmus test you can use to assess an outside-of-class interaction with a student is to ask yourself, "How would I feel if an article describing the interaction appeared the next day in a local newspaper?"

Colleagues at Other Institutions

Pharmacy faculty members have a wonderful opportunity to develop relationships with like-minded colleagues at other institutions. This is especially important if you work at an institution that has few or no colleagues who share your interests.

One of the primary reasons faculty members cite for joining professional organizations is the chance to network with colleagues, which can open doors to many professional collaborations, especially in teaching and scholarship. Joining committees and task forces, being elected to an office, and participating in other activities increases your recognition in the eyes of your colleagues.

Building a positive reputation becomes increasingly important as you move forward in your career. Colleagues from other institutions may be asked to evaluate your performance, especially as part of a promotion or tenure review. Criteria colleagues may use to evaluate your performance will include your contributions to your field and your reputation with your peers.

A final note about relationships: you must prove yourself worthy of your colleagues' respect. It's unrealistic to think they will automatically revere you simply because of your credentials. Everyone you work with, including your students, has gone through trials and tribulations to achieve their current position and level of respect. The respect you offer your colleagues, peers, and students will go a long way toward building their respect for you.

Manage Time and Priorities

Regardless of your field or profession, time management is an essential skill for success in all kinds of endeavors, both at work and at home. Anyone pursuing a career as a faculty member has faced time-management challenges, from getting coursework done to completing research projects and finding time for friends, family, exercise, and sleep. We've all seen examples of people who seem to accomplish their goals and still have time to enjoy themselves, as well as others who always complain that they don't have the time to finish tasks by deadlines, let alone have fun.

The term "time management" is somewhat of a misnomer, in that each day has only 24 hours and you can't do anything to change it. You can save time in different ways, such as eating lunch at your desk rather than going out, but that's merely a matter of finding alternative ways to spend the hours in a day. Time management is really about managing priorities: choosing to spend more time, or at least more quality time, on activities that are important to you.

In some pharmacy practice settings, your priorities are set by the needs of patients. For example, in community and hospital pharmacies, prescription and medication orders are delivered to the pharmacist, who then handles each issue inherent in an order to assure that patients receive the highest quality of care. This process is repeated for each order, and at the end of a work shift, it becomes another pharmacist's responsibility to handle the orders and patient needs.

Managing priorities is different for a faculty member at a college of pharmacy. Work in academia rarely comes as a steady stream of orders. Some things require immediate attention, such as a student stopping by your office with questions about an assignment. Other types of faculty work, such as a research project, can often be carried out when you choose.

Unlike many other types of employee-employer relationships, your department chair or other supervisor will rarely observe your work directly, which gives you great flexibility in how and when you perform it. Most department chairs are more concerned about the quality and quantity of your work (outcomes), and not so much with where and when it was performed (structure and process). Faculty members often cite this freedom as one of the positive aspects of their jobs. But it also brings a great deal of responsibility, in that you are ultimately held accountable to do what is necessary for your success.

Outside of assigning teaching loads and committee service responsibilities, most academic supervisors won't tell you what specific activities you should be doing, such as the topics to cover in a lecture or how to go about conducting a research project. To effectively manage your time, you must set priorities that guide what work needs to be accomplished, by whom, and by when.

A good first step when you start your position is to do a self-assessment. Look closely at how you spend your time and how you handle situations when you have multiple demands. Certainly you've had to manage time and priorities effectively to reach this point in your career, but taking a faculty position creates an entirely new set of time management challenges. A wealth of books, tools, and strategies are available to help; a good source to begin with is the chapter "Time Management/Organizational Skills" by Dana P. Hammer, PhD, in the book *Pharmacy Management: Essentials for all Practice Settings,* which I coedited with Shane P. Desselle, PhD.

Reflect and Plan

Getting a handle on your priorities is an important part of a successful career as a pharmacy faculty member. If your goal is to be promoted or to achieve tenure, your college or university's faculty handbook may help guide you, but only in the most general way—such as the need to achieve excellence in your teaching, scholarship, and service. Your department chair and others you work with may set some specific priorities, such as a particular class or lecture to be taught. But in the end, you, just like every faculty member, are largely on your own to set your professional and personal priorities.

Start with personal reflection to determine what *you* feel is important to achieve. Then develop goals and a road map for how to achieve them. Many faculty members find this process to be much more difficult than it sounds.

It helps if you work with your department chair or other direct supervisor, whose knowledge of institutional values and whose experience coaching other new faculty will be invaluable as you begin to chart your course in academia. Your chair can also work with you to develop a personal strategic plan, similar to a strategic plan developed by any organization, that helps you assess your strengths and weaknesses, recognize opportunities, limit the influence of threats on your success, and create a set of goals and action steps. Hammer's chapter in *Pharmacy Management: Essentials for All Practice Settings,* mentioned above, also includes tips for performing this type of planning.

Documenting your activities is essential to staying on track to achieve your goals. Keep your curriculum vitae (CV) current, just as you did when you began searching for a job. As you start you career as a faculty member, your CV will take on a different purpose—providing a record of your knowledge, skills, interests, and accomplishments as you apply for grants or get more involved in professional organizations.

A Summary of Keys to Success as a Newcomer to Academia

Manage Expectations
- Channel your energy in the right direction.
- Know the balance of teaching, scholarship, and service expected of you.
- Understand your institution's performance expectations.
- Learn how you'll be evaluated for promotion and tenure.

Manage Relationships
- Turn to your department chair first if you have questions.
- Your chair will probably evaluate your performance annually; ask to meet more often to discuss performance expectations and assessment.
- Understand functions of vice chairs and other administrators and build good relationships with them.
- Seek feedback and learn from faculty peers.
- Get to know administrative staff and find out what they can do to help you work more efficiently.
- Build positive relationships with your students and know what to do if problems arise.
- Clearly state the level of performance you expect from students and make sure they understand your assessment approach.
- Set appropriate boundaries with students.
- Develop relationships with colleagues at other institutions.
- Join professional organizations.
- Prove yourself and build a positive reputation.

Manage Time and Priorities
- Recognize that positions in academia come with a great deal of freedom.
- Learn to manage your own time and priorities.
- Assess how you handle competing demands and fine-tune your approach.

Reflect and Plan
- Think about what you feel is important to achieve in your career.
- Develop a road map for achieving your goals.
- Work with your supervisor to help chart your course in academia.

continued on page 111

continued from page 110

- Create a personal strategic plan to assess your strengths and weaknesses, recognize opportunities, sidestep pitfalls, and create goals and action steps.
- Document your activities to stay on track.
- Keep your curriculum vitae and portfolio up to date.

Build Work–Life Balance
- Know what a "balanced life" means for you.
- Look at how colleagues create balance; emulate what works for you.
- Do not adopt unhealthy approaches just because others in the department do.
- Avoid the trap of perfectionism: know when the highest quality is essential and when it isn't.
- Maintain a personal network of family and friends.
- Set a regular work schedule and stick to it.
- Build in time for the other things you want out of life.
- Take care of yourself, including your physical, mental, and spiritual health.

You may also be asked to create a portfolio of your work as evidence of your growth and accomplishments in teaching, scholarship, and service. Portfolios are commonly required of candidates for promotion and tenure. Today, many colleges of pharmacy ask their faculty members to develop a portfolio from the time they start their positions.

Each year you are likely to participate in an annual faculty evaluation process, the details of which vary by institution. You will probably begin by completing a report that compiles and reflects on your accomplishments over the past year. You may also be asked to provide a set of personal goals at the beginning of the process, and then to assess yourself based on the extent to which you achieved these goals over the year. Your department chair and others in your college may take part in evaluating your performance and providing feedback. What you learn from this exercise of reflection and evaluation should help you develop your goals and priorities into the future.

Build Work–Life Balance

No chapter on keys to success as a faculty member would be complete without addressing the need for balance. Obtaining your faculty position should be a means to ends that are meaningful and important to *you,* not an end in itself. A career as a pharmacy faculty member should provide you the flexibility and resources to spend quality time with family and friends, live a lifestyle you enjoy, and make meaningful contributions to students, patients, colleagues, the profession, and society at large.

Look to your colleagues and administrators to see how they balance their personal and professional lives. Think about what makes sense to emulate and what you should avoid. Their actions (and not necessarily their words) often create a culture that new members of the organization feel obliged to follow. Faculty and staff who have unhealthy work habits and wear them as a "badge of courage"—such as working 80 hours a week and never taking vacation or personal days—may create unhealthy expectations for newcomers.

> The work of college faculty members is almost never really "done."

Keep in mind that everyone defines a balanced life differently. What may seem an unhealthy approach for you could actually provide the right balance for a colleague. For example, receiving emails from a colleague at 10 pm may be a sign of excessive work, or it could be that person's way of balancing job demands and time spent with family.

Many pharmacists, regardless of their practice setting, have a tendency toward the work-obsessed "Type A" personality traits, especially perfectionism. Attention to detail is important for performing high-quality work, but trying to attain perfection is time-consuming and draining. Investing additional time to make something "perfect" does not always pay off in the level of quality you'd hoped for. As a new faculty member, it is important to recognize where the highest quality is essential, such as accurate content in a lecture, and where it isn't, such as the first draft of a committee report.

To achieve work–life balance, maintain a personal network of family and friends just as you would maintain your professional network with colleagues. Stay in touch with the people you care about and take time to respond when they reach out to you. Many faculty members use online social networking tools such as Facebook and Twitter to maintain their personal networks. Some even make a conscious decision not to invite coworkers and colleagues into these networks to avoid blurring the lines between their personal and professional lives.

The work of college faculty members is almost never really "done." There is always something else we could be doing, even at the end of the day. An important survival strategy for any pharmacy faculty member is to set a regular work schedule and stick to it as much as possible. You need time to work, but you also need time for all the other things you want out of life.

The most important asset you have in achieving success as a pharmacy faculty member is *you*. Take every step you can to take care of yourself, including your physical, mental, and spiritual health. Many people have a vested interest in seeing you succeed as a faculty member, but you'll never be in a position to effectively help others unless you make your well-being a priority.

Where to Find More Information on Keys to Starting an Academic Career

Promoting Civility in Pharmacy Education
Berger BA, ed. Binghamton, NY: The Haworth Press; 2003
A resource for learning to promote civility in all aspects and settings of pharmacy education, from large lectures to one-on-one interactions with students. Includes specific information regarding incidents of incivility often experienced by new faculty members.

Time Management/Organization Skills
Hammer DP. In: Desselle SP, Zgarrick DP, eds. *Pharmacy Management: Essentials for All Practice Settings.* 2nd ed. New York: McGraw Hill; 2009
Chapter in a pharmacy management textbook that offers time managements strategies and organizational skills useful in a variety of settings and contexts.

Chapter 8

Resources to Help Achieve Success

If you've read this far, you've learned a lot about the challenges and rewards of a career as a faculty member at a college of pharmacy. Deciding to begin a career at a college of pharmacy sets you on a path that most wouldn't trade for any other career in our profession.

Colleges and universities, as well as the profession itself, recognize the importance of supporting the development of their faculty, not only so they can have successful careers, but also so they can contribute to the profession through their teaching, scholarship, and service. To this end, a number of resources are designed to help you achieve success as a faculty member.

College and University Resources

Most colleges and universities have resources and programs to help their faculty transition into academic life and develop their professional careers. Every college of pharmacy offers some degree of support, even if it is simply direction from a department chair and mentoring support from your peers.

Development

Many departments and colleges of pharmacy have formalized their approach to new faculty development. When considering a faculty position, think about which development programs each college offers. Types of programs may include:

- Formal faculty advising and mentoring programs.
- First-year experience seminars.
- Programs that help faculty learn more about specific functions, such as teaching or scholarship.

As a new faculty member, you will probably have
resources available that you can apply toward your
professional development. Once an employment
offer has been extended, new faculty, particularly
in the sciences, often can negotiate for a package of
resources to help start their research, ranging from
laboratory space and equipment to funds for hiring
post docs, graduate students, research assistants,
and others to help move their research forward.

Even clinical faculty should view receiving an offer
as an opportunity to negotiate for resources to
help develop their teaching, practice, and scholarly
pursuits, such as books for their practice site, support for obtaining board certification, or attendance
at a program to help build key skills. Don't be afraid
to ask for resources; you're unlikely to get them
otherwise.

> Deciding to begin a career at a college of pharmacy sets you on a path that most wouldn't trade for any other career in our profession.

At the same time, be realistic in your expectations and don't ask for things that
either aren't typically needed by others performing similar roles or available
at your type of institution. The resources you request are granted with the
expectation that you will use them to develop and advance your career and
bring something back to your college or university, such as research grants,
publications, or publicity for the good work you are doing. The greater the level
of resources provided when you begin, the greater the expectations placed on
you for performance at some later point.

Many departments and colleges provide faculty an annual professional development stipend. These are usually relatively small, ranging from several hundred
to several thousand dollars per year, and are meant to allow faculty to join
professional organizations, subscribe to journals, purchase books and other
materials related to their teaching and research, and perhaps attend a professional conference. Your department or college may have rules on how these
funds can be spent. For example, priority may be given to colleagues who will
be presenting posters or papers at a conference. Make it a point to ask about
the availability and use of these funds during the negotiation process.

Teaching and Learning

A number of universities, recognizing that newly hired faculty are relatively
inexperienced teachers, have developed centers for teaching and learning
or for educational technology to promote learning about effective pedagogy.

Because educational technology is advancing rapidly and computers, the Internet, wireless networks, and new software allow learning to take place anywhere, anytime, educational technology centers help faculty integrate the latest tools into their classes.

Younger faculty who grew up with online technologies may be more comfortable with them than more seasoned faculty members are, which might give you opportunities to take the lead on integrating newer technologies into your teaching and to help other faculty make better use of them, too.

Other Options

Most colleges and universities offer other resources designed to help their faculty succeed, such as an office of research and sponsored programs to develop institutional policies and procedures pertaining to research and administering the institutional review board. These offices provide other assistance, too, which is important because developing as a researcher is essential for earning promotion and tenure at many universities. For example, they may provide guidance in obtaining grants, usually by informing researchers of opportunities for funding (requests for proposals) and helping to improve faculty grant-writing skills. It's essential that new faculty learn about the policies and procedures regarding research and other scholarly activities and, whenever possible, take advantage of programs offered by the university.

Professional Organization Resources

Many professional organizations offer resources to assist members involved in education and research. These groups recognize the importance of supporting college faculty. In turn, faculty members benefit by having opportunities to learn about advances in their fields, a forum to present their research and other scholarly work, grant support for their research and teaching activities, leadership development, and the chance to network with peers in their fields.

American Association of Colleges of Pharmacy

AACP (www.aacp.org) is the professional organization most closely aligned with the needs of colleges of pharmacy and their faculty members. It provides countless resources to faculty at all stages of their careers, ranging from student pharmacists considering careers in academia to faculty members just starting out and experienced faculty and administrators.

As with many professional organizations, AACP enables members to join affinity groups based on scientific or clinical interests (similar to departments in most colleges), functions at their schools (faculty, deans, and other administrators), or specialized interests, such as assessment, curricular development, educational technology, and admissions. Each group gives its members opportunities to learn more about their fields and interests, to present scholarly work related to pharmacy education, and to take advantage of leadership opportunities in the group.

AACP sponsors an annual and an interim meeting open to the general membership, as well as conferences aimed at the needs of specific groups, such as experiential education personnel or development officers. AACP also offers programs to help faculty and administrators build their skills. Among these are the Teacher's Seminar, Education Scholar Program, and Academic Leadership Fellows Program. Finally, AACP publishes the *American Journal of Pharmaceutical Education* (*AJPE*), a leading peer-reviewed journal in pharmacy education.

American College of Clinical Pharmacy

ACCP (www.accp.com) offers a wide variety of resources for faculty members, primarily aimed at clinical practitioners and researchers. Like most organizations, AACP has affinity groups based on clinical specialty and functions, as well as educational programming through both conferences and educational materials.

Among its educational materials is the Pharmacotherapy Self-Assessment Program (PSAP), which many board-certified pharmacotherapy specialists and subspecialists use to keep abreast of new clinical developments. It has also developed the ACCP Academy, which consists of four tracks of professional development programming in leadership and management, research and scholarship, teaching and learning, and clinical practice advancement.

Of particular interest to clinical researchers is ACCP's Research Institute (www.accpri.org), which provides a variety of development resources including the Focused Investigator Training Program (FIT) and Practice-Based Research Network (PBRN).

Other Key Groups

Many other organizations offer resources for pharmacy faculty members and educators, including affinity groups:

- American Association of Pharmaceutical Scientists (AAPS) www.aapspharmaceutica.com
- American Pharmacists Association (APhA) www.pharmacist.com
- American Society of Consultant Pharmacists (ASCP) www.ascp.com

- American Society of Health-System Pharmacists (ASHP) www.ashp.org
- International Pharmaceutical Federation (FIP) www.fip.org
- National Association of Chain Drug Stores (NACDS) www.nacds.org
- National Community Pharmacists Association (NCPA) www.ncpanet.org

General Academic Support Resources

Faculty of all kinds, including those not affiliated with a college, university, or professional association, can take advantage of a number of resources. For example, the first issue of the journal *Currents in Pharmacy Teaching and Learning* was dedicated to clinical faculty development, and each issue contains helpful overviews and insights. Books are also available to help faculty, including *Handbook for Pharmacy Education: Getting Adjusted as a New Pharmacy Faculty Member* by Shane Desselle and Dana Hammer, and *What Matters in Teaching and Learning in Pharmacy Education* by Lynne Sylvia and Judith Barr.

Many resources are not necessarily specific to pharmacy education, but provide helpful insights about the general development of a new faculty member. One of the best is *The Teaching Professor* (www.teachingprofessor.com), which started as a monthly newsletter and now also includes a website with blogs on a variety of teaching topics as well as an annual conference. *The Teaching Professor* is structured to provide short articles based on faculty members' experiences of what works and what doesn't in their own teaching. It is a very easy newsletter to read and is often a source of inspiration to new faculty when the going gets rough.

> The greater the level of resources provided when you begin, the greater the expectations placed on you for performance at some later point.

Many books have been developed to help faculty develop their teaching skills; a particularly helpful one is *Learner-Centered Teaching: Five Key Changes to Practice* by Maryellen Weimer. Two that stand out on the subject of developing as a new faculty member are *Advice for New Faculty Members* by Robert Boice and *Mentor in a Manual: Climbing the Academic Ladder to Tenure* by A. Clay Schoenfeld and Robert Magnan. Both take a practical approach to describing the opportunities and challenges inherent in becoming a college faculty member.

Final Thoughts on Getting Started

After reading this book, you probably have many thoughts and new perspectives about getting started as a pharmacy faculty member. On the one hand, you've learned that the task of being a faculty member entails much more than may be apparent to the outside observer, and that colleges and universities are complex organizations that can both enhance and impede one's professional development. In this book, I've tried to give you a realistic, rather than idealistic, viewpoint on faculty life to better prepare you for challenges that lie ahead.

On the other hand, you've learned about the many rewards of being a faculty member. I know of no other career that offers such flexibility and autonomy in your professional life while allowing you to have a profound effect on the lives of others. I hope my descriptions of the ways you have freedom and influence in colleges of pharmacy motivate you to achieve your own measure of success as you get started as a pharmacy faculty member.

Where to Find More Information on Resources to Help Achieve Success

Advice for New Faculty Members: Nihil Nimus
Boice R. Needham Heights, Mass: Allyn & Bacon; 2000
A general guide for new faculty members in all academic fields. Emphasizes the importance of moderation in approaching the various aspects of faculty work, while describing the differences between new faculty members who struggle and those who succeed in their roles.

American Journal of Pharmaceutical Education
www.ajpe.org
The official publication of the American Association of Colleges of Pharmacy, this peer-reviewed journal publishes original research, descriptions of innovations in teaching, instructional design and assessment, and viewpoints pertaining to pharmacy education.

continued on page 121

continued from 120

Currents in Pharmacy Teaching and Learning
www.elsevier.com
A peer-reviewed pharmacy education journal published by Elsevier that focuses on reports of innovative teaching and learning strategies, skills development, outcomes assessment, curricular revision, and practical tips from seasoned educators.

Handbook for Pharmacy Educators: Getting Adjusted as a New Pharmacy Faculty Member
Desselle SP, Hammer DP. Binghamton, NY: The Haworth Press; 2002
Describes the experiences of six junior faculty members as they start their experiences in academic pharmacy.

Learner-Centered Teaching: Five Key Changes to Practice
Weimer M. San Francisco: Jossey-Bass; 2002
Explains how college and university faculty can implement learner-centered strategies to enhance the student experience in the classroom and improve knowledge retention.

Mentor in a Manual: Climbing the Academic Ladder to Tenure, 3rd ed.
Schoenfeld AC, Magnan R. Madison, Wis: Atwood Publications; 2004
A commonly referenced guide to the roles of teaching, scholarship, and service at various stages of the tenure-track process.

Teaching Professor
www.teachingprofessor.com
A website, newsletter, and blog containing words of wisdom from experienced educators in all fields. Also sponsors an annual conference dedicated to educating, engaging and inspiring faculty in teaching and learning.

What Matters in Teaching and Learning in Pharmacy Education
Sylvia L, Barr J., eds. New York: Jossey-Bass; 2010
Guide to effective teaching and learning strategies specific to pharmacy education.

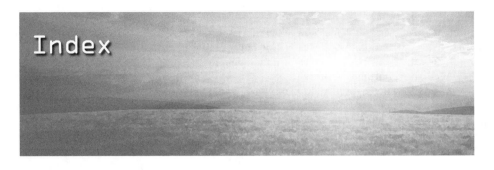

Index

Note: Page numbers followed by *b, f,* and *t* indicate text boxes, figures, and tables, respectively.

A

B

C

E

F

W